REENGAGE
WITH LIFE & FAMILY

HOW TREATING HEARING LOSS
can change your **life**, maintain your **independence**,
and may **reduce** your risk of **dementia**

DR. DANA DAY, AUD
DR. KEITH N. DARROW, PHD

EIA MEDIA GROUP

Reengage With Life & Family: How treating hearing loss can change your life,
maintain your independence, and may reduce your risk of dementia
— by Dr. Dana Day, AuD, and Dr. Keith N. Darrow, PhD

Project Director: Jared M. Brader, MBA
Editor: Kelly Martin
Graphics: Steve Ruesch
Cover & Interior Design: Five J's Design, FiveJsDesign.com

First Printing: June 2019

ISBN: 978-1-7958-3367-7

To my dad who taught me the value of hard work,
and my mother who taught me the value of a kind word,
gentle touch, and art of listening.

To my patients who have entrusted themselves and the
hearing and balance healthcare to me, I am humbled
and hope I made a difference, if only a small one, in your lives.

Most of all my children, who bring me such joy
and inspire me to be better each day.

— D.D.

Dad, I miss you.

Laura, I love you.

EMC^D, I love you even more.

Jared, Thank you.

— K.D.

TABLE OF CONTENTS

REENGAGE
WITH LIFE & FAMILY

A NOTE FROM DR. DANA DAY

I WANT TO CONGRATULATE YOU FOR BEING COURAGEOUS

and raising your hand to start the medical treatment of your hearing loss. Yes, I said *medical* treatment of your hearing loss. While this can seem daunting, it really doesn't need to be. We will walk you through the process in this book—from why your hearing is so important, who you should see, what to expect, the long-term cost of *not* treating your hearing loss, and so much more.

You will understand why treating your hearing loss can change your life and may reduce your risk of dementia. This is not just "pie in the sky"; Dr. Darrow and I will present the research studies supporting why the medical treatment of hearing loss is so important. We will discuss the co-morbidities of hearing loss and disease state conditions such as diabetes, heart disease, kidney disease, balance issues, fall risk, and more.

You will also learn why the medical treatment of hearing loss is *not* your father's hearing aid and why it is so important to know the difference between technology that allows for more clarity of speech vs. a device that simply makes all sound louder.

So please take the time to read our book; highlight, underline, and write your questions in the margins of the pages. When you are ready to say, "Yes, I am ready to medically treat my hearing loss," we are *hear for you.*

Yours in better hearing,
DANA L. DAY, AuD, CCC-A, MBA

ABOUT THE AUTHORS

DR. DANA DAY, AUD

is the founder and current Director of Audiology for Arizona Balance & Hearing, and she is leading the movement to medically treat hearing loss in the greater Phoenix area. By working alongside her team of hearing health care specialists, including Neuroscientist Dr. Keith Darrow, Brain Fitness Specialists, NeuroTechnology™ Treatment Specialists, and her entire patient experience team, Dr. Day is able to focus on medically treating *your* hearing loss, tinnitus, and balance disorders and the associated cognitive impacts.

Dr. Day is instinctually described as an 'Innovator' by Kathy Kolbe, the world's leading authority on human instincts. Dr. Day continues to defy convention, challenge her team at Arizona Balance & Hearing, and make the world a better place by improving the lives of her patients each and every day.

Dr. Day began her training in Germany at the 2nd General Regional Hospital serving our brave men and women in uniform and NATO Troops throughout Europe. Dr. Day was instrumental in the development of several balance and concussion centers throughout Phoenix, including the Barrow Neurological Institute, where she furthered her knowledge on how the brain and hearing work together.

Dr. Day's impact on our organization, the profession, and the world includes:

- being trained by Dr. Keith Darrow, the only Harvard and M.I.T. Trained Neuroscientist and Audiologist in the world, as part of the Excellence in Audiology Movement which focuses your hearing loss treatment on sound medical and neuroscience necessity rather than traditional hearing aids;

- restoring hearing clarity for thousands of individuals in the greater Phoenix area with hearing loss just like yours;

- being a leader in public seminars and symposiums in the Phoenix area where she educates our community on hearing loss and dementia, tinnitus, and balance disorders;

- teaching the next generation of Doctors of Audiology at Arizona State University;

- being a rising star amongst her peers and a leading change agent amongst her fellow Doctors as a Fellow of the American Academy of Audiology;

- her practice being a teaching and training facility for the next generation of hearing health care providers from around the country;

- her articles being included in *The Hearing Journal* and American Tinnitus Association periodicals; and

- volunteering at Hospice of the Valley, providing care to their hearing-impaired patients in the late season of their lives.

DR. KEITH N. DARROW, PHD

is an expert in Speech and Hearing Bioscience and Technology with a doctoral degree from the joint Massachusetts Institute of Technology (M.I.T) and Harvard Medical School program. He is a former Clinical Professor at Northeastern University (Boston, MA) and is currently a tenured professor at Worcester State University.

Dr. Darrow's clinical experience is vast and includes a clinical fellowship at the Department of Otolaryngology at Brigham and Women's Hospital (Boston, MA) and a trainingship at the Audiology Department in the East Orange (NJ) Veterans Association Hospital. He is the owner of the Hearing and Balance Centers of New England and founder of the Healthy Hearing Foundation of New England, as well as a board member of the Sound of Life Foundation (both non-profit organizations dedicated to providing education and hearing health care for those in need). He was recently named the Director of Audiology Research at Intermountain Audiology and has chosen to lead the Excellence In Audiology movement across the country.

Dr. Darrow is a nationally recognized speaker, trainer, and researcher and has been conducting research at the Massachusetts Eye and Ear Infirmary for over fifteen years. His publications and research have been cited over 550 times. On a personal note, Dr. Darrow and his wife Laura have three children (Ella, Mae and Charlie) who love to ski and travel to National Parks together. He also serves on the board of directors for the Worcester County Reserve Deputy Sheriffs Association and provides countless hours of volunteer service in his communities.

PREFACE

TODAY, APPROXIMATELY 48 MILLION PEOPLE in the United States are suffering from hearing loss. Yet, nearly 40 million of them go without treatment. Hence, the reason I wrote this book.

- *Do you want to remain independent and live an active life as you age?*

- *Did you know that hearing problems, even at the mildest stage, can lead to social isolation and increase the risk of dementia?*

- *Do you or a loved one have impaired hearing?*

Hi, I'm Dr. Keith N. Darrow, Ph.D. CCC-A, a trained Neuroscientist and practicing Clinical Audiologist. If you or a loved one has answered yes to any of the above questions, I encourage you to read this book and learn how you can live a better, more active, more engaged, and healthier life as you age. For over twenty years, I have been helping my patients, and their loved ones, break free of their hearing loss and live an active, engaged life—free of the worry, stress, and medical consequences of untreated hearing loss.

Hearing is what connects us to others. Hearing is a requirement for every personal and professional relationship we have; it is the building block of communication.

Hearing is also one of the major senses; in fact, I believe it is the single most important sense we have. While hearing certainly plays a major role in our fight or flight, prey vs. predator, and history as human beings, hearing today has the important role of keeping us communicating and connected with the world around us—at home, at work, and in our community. To further support my claim that hearing is the single most important sense we have, I offer the fact that the organ of hearing, the cochlea (AKA the inner ear), is embedded deep in the hardest bone in the entire human body, the petrous portion of the temporal bone (i.e. petrous means "stone/rock")—thus providing our organ of hearing significant protection.

I have put together this book to help you understand the dire consequences of untreated hearing loss and to introduce you to how today's medical options for treating hearing loss can not only help improve hearing, but also improve cognitive function, decrease your risk of developing dementia, depression, and falling, while also increasing your physical activity, and helping you live a happier and healthier lifestyle as you actively age.

Hearing loss has been listed by the Department of Health and Human Services as the third most common chronic health condition affecting seniors. *Third!* Hearing loss is estimated to affect nearly 50% of adults between the age of sixty to seventy years young, nearly 2/3 of adults between seventy to eighty years young, and the numbers only go up from there! As we live longer and science continues to increase life expectancy, we need to be best prepared to deal with this debilitating disorder and understand how it can impact our lives.

My journey up to this point has been filled with over twenty years of experience—from student to clinician to scientist to college professor and back to clinician and patient advocate. I was lucky to discover what I love to do in life, and as a result I have the good fortune to work with patients and their families every day as they embark on the journey of improved hearing and clarity.

While my elementary and high school performance wasn't much to speak of (in fact, I was dismissed from high school twice—but that is a story for a different day!), once I found my path of helping people understand and improve the process of communication in their daily lives, it all became incredibly easy for me.

In fact, I was on the Dean's List nearly every semester in college, graduated in the top 5% of my Clinical Audiology Program in New

York City, and went on to be the only practicing audiologist to complete a Doctoral Degree in the Neuroscience track at M.I.T. and Harvard Medical School.

As a trained Neuroscientist, expert in Speech and Hearing Bioscience and Technology, and a practicing clinical audiologist, I have a unique perspective on how the brain works and how hearing relates to overall health, well-being, and cognitive function. I also understand how treating hearing loss *early* (even before it becomes a problem that you and everybody around you can notice) significantly impacts your overall health and cognitive function and how it may significantly reduce your risk of developing dementia.

I believe that I am blessed to have the capability of transforming lives and families every single day. Treating hearing loss is not magic—it is the perfect mix of science and experience, which allows myself and my team to use advances in medical treatment of hearing loss, NeuroTechnology™, to stimulate the brain, improve cognitive function and mental health, and help adults remain independent. And the best part—it is simple for patients to manage and it's affordable!

INTRODUCTION

The Top 5 Reasons People Avoid Seeing a Hearing Care Specialist

MY NAME IS DR. KEITH N. DARROW, and I'm a trained Neuroscientist and Clinical Audiologist! When people hear what I do for a living, they almost automatically…wince! They try not to be too obvious about it. (Hey, I have feelings, too!). It's okay; I'm used to it. The fact is, the less you know about audiology and treating hearing loss, the more reason you have to be afraid of it. Once upon a time, audiology meant one thing: big, heavy, ugly "beige bananas" to be worn on your ear to make sounds louder.

They were hard to put on, hard to make adjustments to, and, frankly, they were pretty terrible at doing anything other than making all sounds louder…this includes speech, background noise, loud ventilation machines, dogs barking, plates clanging, etc.!

For the majority of patients, wearing an old fashioned hearing aid meant avoiding certain social situations, restaurants, family gatherings, playing with grandchildren, etc. Many people still cling to the unfounded notion that all hearing aids are created equal and perform the same way they did back in 1982!

The fact of the matter is that audiology and the clinical science of treating hearing loss is more than just hearing aids. How much more? *Audiology and the medical treatment of hearing loss is devoted to restoring an individual's clarity, restoring personal independence, improving cognitive function and mental health, and addressing the cognitive aspects of hearing loss that can increase the risk of developing dementia.*

Maintaining proper hearing and cognitive health has a significant impact on an individual's life—including all of his or her family, friends, and community members. Properly stimulating cognitive function and maintaining connections from the ear to the brain goes a long way in keeping a patient mentally competent, helping the patient remain autonomous, and helping keep at bay the mind-robbing diseases associated with cognitive decline (i.e. Alzheimer's). Treating hearing loss is a wonderful investment with life-long returns, and yet people still fear walking into a hearing health care provider's office for one simple reason—fear of the unknown!

Hey—it's okay to be worried about the unknown. We all have our reasons for avoiding the doctor. For example, I underwent aggressive management of atypical moles on my body (to avoid potentially pre-cancerous melanoma). I was scared. I avoided starting the treatment for several years. Until I realized that enough is enough…and I had my family bugging me to do something before it was too late. Starting treatment was the right thing to do, and while it was impossible to know the results had I not started treatment…the potential is there for me not having ever had the opportunity to write this book (if you catch my drift!).

For many, visiting a Doctor of Audiology is accompanied by many fears and anxieties. And for each patient, the experience is personal. There are reasons that patients typically wait seven years before being seen by a Doctor of Audiology and beginning treatment of their hearing loss. This list, *Top 5 Reasons People Avoid Seeing a Hearing Care Specialist,* has the most common conversations I have had with patients over the past twenty years about what took them so long to come in to my office.

While you may not place treating potentially pre-cancerous moles and treating hearing loss on the same level of importance, I promise that by the time you are done with this book you will understand why that premise is absolutely wrong and how the consequences of untreated hearing loss can negatively impact every part of your life, even rendering you dependent on others and at a significantly increased risk of developing dementia.

REASON #1 — The Patient Already Knows the Diagnosis Before He or She Ever Steps Foot in the Door.

Individuals with hearing loss have a tendency to wait nearly seven years before raising their hand and admitting they have a problem. Or perhaps it takes a family member nearly seven years to push his or her loved one through our office door! Either way, seven seems to be the "unlucky" number—I say "unlucky" because chances are very high that by the seventh year of experiencing the symptoms of hearing loss, significant damage has been done to the auditory system, which can lower treatment outcomes. I try to explain to all of my patients that hearing loss is a progressive degenerative disorder with neurologic involvement which undoubtedly requires early intervention. In lay terms, that simply means that your hearing will continue to degrade as you age, and the key to maintaining clarity and a higher level of hearing function (i.e. hearing in noisy environments) is to *catch it early and treat it early.*

I have empathy for the new patient who comes to my office to get his or her first hearing evaluation since grade school because I know, as does the patient, what the results will likely be. It is very brave for a patient to knowingly enter a medical office with the understanding that he or she is likely to receive the diagnosis of progressive degenerative age-related hearing loss. And that this disorder is neither reversible, nor is there a cure. However, there are restorative treatments available that can help the patient stay connected at home, at work, and in the community, and that can help stimulate the brain, improve cognitive function, and even reduce the risk of developing dementia (more on the connections of hearing loss and dementia later in the book!).

REASON #2 — The Patient is Not Sure of His or Her Insurance Coverage for the Procedures and Treatments Involved with Hearing Loss.

Regardless of when you read this book and which administration is running our country, insurance is a complex world to attempt to muddle through, and when it comes to hearing health care coverage, it can be even more murky. BUT…nearly every insurance company I have come across allows for coverage of one hearing evaluation per year by a trained hearing health care specialist (and more testing can be covered if medically necessary, i.e. if the patient notices a significant sudden change in hearing). A hearing evaluation is often considered "preventative" and, in many cases, does not require a referral from your physician.

While it is nearly impossible to speak for every patient and every insurance plan, this is intended to help ease the stress of navigating the process of hearing health care coverage. In fact, I believe any reputable hearing health care practice will have a deep understanding of the insurance regulations in its area and will be able to readily answer any questions you may have about your insurance coverage—or at least be willing to help you find the answer.

In my twenty years of experience in the hearing health care field, I have watched first hand as patient benefits for treatment of hearing loss have evolved—fortunately, in a direction that benefits the patient. Yes, medical treatment of your hearing loss may have an out-of-pocket cost associated with it, but I have seen insurance cover anywhere from 10% to 100% of the costs. And even if you were in the position of having

0% insurance coverage, treating hearing loss can be affordable—and you will learn throughout this book that treating hearing loss is truly priceless and can hardly be assigned a monetary value.

REASON #3 — Patients are Afraid of Being Sold Something.

It's like magic—once you turn the respectful age of sixty, you notice that the content of your mailbox seems to change. Nearly every week, perhaps a few times a week, you are "blessed" (I'm being sarcastic!) to have a full mailbox (both your physical and electronic mailbox) with literature about "essential vitamins for seniors," "how to choose the right assisted living residence," "how to invest your retirement money," "join AARP," and "which digital technology widget is best for your hearing loss." Somewhere along the line, hearing health care started down the dangerous road of becoming a retail transaction. Heck, I've even seen some hearing widgets sold at big-box retailers and chain pharmacies… although I don't know who would ever consider buying medical treatment for a progressive degenerative disorder alongside a giant vat of peanut butter! Like I ask my patients: *"Would you get your colonoscopy performed at one of the big-box chains? NO…so why would you treat your hearing loss there?"* I don't blame the patient for sometimes entering the office thinking he/she is going to be "sold" something.

My best advice is to steer clear of anybody trying to sell you something. If we go back to Reason #1 above, the patient is likely already nervous because he or she knows the medical diagnosis before ever even stepping foot in the office. Combine that with the fear of "being sold something" and that makes for a pretty nervous patient with his or her guard up.

Unfortunately, much of modern medicine is turning into a commercial advertisement seen on TV that marginalizes the process of treating a medical disorder; and hearing health care is not immune to this. In my office, and the Excellence in Audiology member-clinics across the country, our belief is in the medical evaluation and treatment of hearing loss.

I believe strongly that the proper medical treatment of hearing loss is best left to the clinicians specially trained to understand, diagnose, and treat your hearing loss.

REASON #4 — The Cost.

Actual Cost

We all know somebody, perhaps a family member or a friend, who has spent a significant amount of money on a hearing aid gizmo only to use it as a paperweight or to leave it in his or her sock drawer. And the reason is because the glorified over-priced amplifier that he or she purchased was never truly designed to improve hearing or clarity—it was designed to just make sounds louder. This truly angers me, and while I do believe that the patient plays a significant role in his or her health care decisions and follow-up care, the health care provider also must have a significant responsibility to the patient—even after the patient has left the office.

I have heard many horror stories about patients spending upwards of $10,000.00 on a pair of hearing aid gizmos—YIKES! More often than not, this very high retail transaction very likely took place in one of the chain hearing aid sales shops (i.e. the "Miracle Hearing" and "Bellstone" shops. FYI the real names of these retail establishments have been altered in an attempt to reduce my chances of being sued!). And, sadly, all the patient got in return for his or her money was a hearing aid amplifier capable of making things louder.

When a practice and the providers are committed to the medical treatment of hearing loss, you can trust that you are in good hands. I believe that a hearing specialist must meet the strict standards required of Excellence in Audiology member-clinics and follow the medical model of treating hearing loss.

I have always believed that the patient needs options to help him or her invest in proper hearing health care. A reputable audiology practice understands that for some people, the upfront investment in hearing healthcare can be prohibitive. Patients must be provided with options. All Excellence In Audiology member-clinics will offer TreatmentFi™, a simple, affordable way to treat hearing loss. This program is sub-scription-based and provides access to affordable hearing health care without compromise. The TreatmentFi™ program offers a lifetime warranty for all technology (including loss of devices), complete access to supplies and batteries, all treatment and diagnostic appointments, and no-cost automatic upgrades of NeuroTechnology™ as hearing and cognitive needs change.

Hidden Cost

What about the cost of **_not_** treating hearing loss? While research has yet to make the definitive finding that hearing loss can *cause* dementia (causality is often difficult in clinical science), the evidence that the re-lationship exists is overwhelming. Even more important is the mount-ing evidence that treating hearing loss may significantly reduce the risk of developing dementia.

Every day, 10,000 people turn sixty-five years young. This trend is expected to continue for at least the next fifteen years. And it is almost a guarantee that over the next fifteen years, science will continue to reduce the mortality rate and increase the average life expectancy. As a result, our health care system will be pushed to its capacity to deal with diseases such as cancer, diabetes, cardiovascular disease, etc. Per-haps the most prevalent, most costly, and most disabling of all diseas-es we will see sharply rise over the ensuing decades is dementia—the mind-robbing mental disease that interrupts and interferes with every aspect of life. Dementia is ___not___ a normal part of aging.

Every three to four seconds, another patient is diagnosed with dementia. Rates of dementia are estimated to triple in the next thirty years. Unlike the other diseases listed above, a physical body with dementia is estimated to outlive the individual's mental capabilities by ten or more years! It is estimated that the average cost, per family, to manage the medical treatment and care of a loved one with dementia can exceed $57,000.00 per year.

There is no cure for this catastrophic disease, but there are treatments available, including several ways to decrease your risk of developing dementia. **In fact, a study published in The Lancet journal indicated that the treatment of hearing loss as the single most effective means of preventing dementia.**

I encourage you to read my report detailing "9 Key Lifestyle Tips to Reduce the Risk of Developing Dementia." This report can be found at *www.ExcellenceInAudiology.org.*

REASON #5 — Everybody *HATES* Hearing Aids.

Let's be honest. Everybody hates hearing aids. In fact, when you make a reference to old-fashioned volume-enhancing hearing aids, I think you could go so far as to say "Some hearing aids suck!" There you have it—I said it! I've been working with hearing-impaired patients for nearly twenty years and although my patients love improved hearing, they hate their hearing aids. I don't see a reason to tip-toe around this subject or ignore the fact that patients generally do not like using hearing aids. Nobody wants a medical disorder that requires physically tethering a device to his or her body to treat the medical condition. People who wear glasses do not actually *want* to wear glasses (although I do know some people who wear non-prescriptive glasses because they feel that they look "cool"). I remember growing up in a time where people who wore glasses were sometimes referred to as "four-eyes" or other derogatory terms—fortunately glasses are now commonplace for people of all ages. I know that in the next few years, I will likely begin to hold the restaurant menu farther and farther away from my face in a dimly lit restaurant and when that happens I will need to invest in the proper treatment of visual impairment—whether I want to wear glasses or not.

For some people, hearing aids carry the stigma of meaning "I'm old and ready to die." And nearly every day I see a patient try and talk him- or herself out of investing in hearing health care treatment because "eh, I won't be around much longer anyway." My response is always the same: if you live for three more days, three more months, three more years, or even thirty more years (which is not unreasonable to expect from my fifty-eight year young patients), isn't it worth wanting to hear and understand everything and everyone else in your life? I also point out to patients that they will appear to look much older if they continue to say "What?" or "Huh?" all the time or, perhaps even worse, start to isolate themselves from the conversation.

I get it, and I respect that patients don't want to use a hearing aid, whatever the reason may be. Any reputable hearing health care provider will realize this, also, and understand the difference between traditional hearing aids and advanced NeuroTechnology™. Features in NeuroTechnology™ are specifically designed to treat the medical condition of hearing loss, improve cognitive function, and improve overall quality of life. As an added benefit, NeuroTechnology™ is incredibly discrete and comes in several invisible styles (more on invisible hearing-loss treatment options later in the book).

PART 1

FINDING A HEARING HEALTH CARE SPECIALIST

QUESTION #1

Why is hearing so important?

I believe most people can relate to my story: I watched my grand-mother degrade as she crossed over from her seventies to her eighties. As she got older, her hearing got worse—and as the hearing got worse, her cognitive abilities declined. As a result, our ability to communicate with her was significantly strained. This is when I first knew that hearing loss must be correlated to cognitive decline (AKA dementia).

Communication is truly the basic building block of every relationship we have at work, at home with our loved ones, with our children, etc. Communication is a vital part of establishing and maintaining relationships. Watching my grandmother decline helped push me to be a better student, a better teacher, and a better clinician. When I decided to veer from clinical audiology for several years to focus on my studies at M.I.T. and Harvard Medical School, I decided to point my efforts at understanding the neuroscience of how we hear at the most basic level—from vibrating molecules of air to neural activity in the brain. Armed with this knowledge, I have been able to advance my patients' care to the highest level and help to set standards for testing and treatment protocol used in clinics across the country.

QUESTION #2

What are some of the early signs of hearing loss, and when should I see a hearing specialist?

Hearing loss is typically a slow, gradual onset disorder that silently (pardon the pun) affects the individual. The most common symptoms experienced by most (perhaps not all) patients are difficulty hearing in background noise, tinnitus, and thinking most people mumble or speak softly! Most people who experience the initial symptoms of hearing loss do not even realize it is happening. It is far easier to blame the acoustics of the room, the volume of the background noise, or the person speaking (i.e. "they mumble") than it is to accept that it's your hearing that is lacking. It is also difficult for many patients to rationalize the need for medical treatment of hearing loss because in some (ideal listening) situations (i.e. sitting at a table one-on-one in a perfectly quiet environment) may not be much of a challenge. But the truth is…

A Mild Hearing Loss is a Major Problem!

The first symptom of hearing loss for most patients is difficulty hearing in complex listening environments. If you take the time to reflect truly and deeply on your communication breakdown, I believe you will begin to recognize some of the initial symptoms of hearing loss. Are you having any difficulty when there are a few people at the kitchen table? Or when the kids come over? Or when communicating with your grandchildren? Or when you are at a social gathering (i.e. sharing a meal with friends and you can't seem to follow the conversation, yet all the other people seem to be enjoying themselves and following the conversation)? It is in these types of scenarios when hearing loss can really start to rear its ugly head and you realize that you are no longer an active part of the conversation. The result is a slow retraction from contributing to the conversation because you may feel embarrassed, and thus you continue to further isolate yourself and find yourself not truly engaging in conversations and relationships. And this is how even a mild hearing loss can really begin to impact your quality of life and relationships with others.

In addition to the importance of maintaining an active, engaged life with family and friends, early treatment of mild hearing loss is important for maintaining proper brain health. Simply put: Hearing Care is Health Care™. Your hearing drives your conception of everything and everybody around you; thus, hearing is essentially driving cognition at all times. It's driving memory. It's driving your image of the environment around you. You don't turn hearing on or off; you can't close your ears like you can close your eyes. There really isn't a sense or portion of your brain that isn't connected to your auditory system.

And I believe this speaks to how important hearing is to live and to thrive. We are bombarded with sound at all times and the brain is constantly, in real-time, making decisions as to whether or not certain sounds are important, trying to figure out how to categorize the sound and if it is important to store away and remember it for reference at a later date. A mild hearing loss can take away significant portions of the auditory world around you—and is likely the reason behind why patients with untreated hearing loss are at a significantly higher risk of experiencing a devastating fall.

The lack of cognitive stimulation that accompanies even a mild hearing loss is also associated with cognitive decline and dementia. Reports from Johns Hopkins Medical Center (and others) indicate that a <u>mild</u> hearing loss can increase the risk of developing dementia by 200% (up to a 500% increase for those with a severe hearing loss).

Like every major medical condition, the key to successful management of the disorder is early intervention. ***"Catch it early and treat it early!"***

QUESTION #3

Why, and how, should I choose a specialist for my hearing loss treatment?

I get this question so often that I developed a Top 10 List (although it's not nearly as fun as David Letterman's Top 10 Lists). This list can help a patient understand "why" they need to choose a specialist and "how" to choose the right specialist to trust with the treatment of their hearing loss. For a more detailed report than what is provided here, visit *www.ExcellenceInAudiology.org* for the full report.

The Top 10 Things You Must Know before Choosing Your Hearing Health Care Provider

❶ Is He or She a Specialist?

Hearing health care consists of both Audiologist and Hearing Instrument Specialist; both working towards the same goal—to help more people struggling with hearing loss. Audiologists are clinically trained hearing health care specialists that take on several extra years of training in order to provide the most thorough diagnostic evaluation and complete the most comprehensive treatment plans aimed at restoring hearing clarity. Hearing Instrument Specialist are trained and licensed professionals that dispense hearing aids. These hearing health care providers perform auditory rehabilitation, which is likely to include the use of NeuroTechnology™ that provides proper stimulation to the auditory system. This is a fancy way to describe how we normalize the way our brains process the incoming sounds in order to achieve maximum clarity, especially in background noise. While there are many hearing health care providers, less than 2% of all audiologists are Excellence in Audiology members.

As the leader of the Excellence In Audiology movement, I don't just treat hearing problems; I also teach clinicians across the country how to become better hearing health care providers. In fact, I have shared my knowledge and taught hundreds of hearing health care specialists throughout the world. By teaching and interacting with many clinicians, I am able to stay at the cutting edge with the best treatment options for my patients.

Another sign of a great specialist is he or she can show you a before and after of a similar case that he or she has previously helped. We know all ears are different, but with the 100,000+ ears our member-clinics have restored clarity to, we can show you a similar case to your specific hearing situation.

❷ Does the Hearing Health Care Provider Have a Medical Office (or a Sales Office)?

In the audiology world, it is not hard to open up shop on a shoe-string budget and call yourself a specialist. When you are searching for a provider, make sure you understand the clinician's credentials and medical affiliations. Often times, smaller offices with limited staff and audiology providers are somewhat limited in their service offerings and stability.

If you find a hearing care provider with the best credentials and an office that is inviting and in a medical setting, you have found a specialist who understands the importance of hearing health care and will be around for years to come to help you and your family best understand and address your hearing needs. For a list of Excellence In Audiology member-clinics, visit *www.ExcellenceInAudiology.org.*

Excellence in Audiology member-clinics are located across the country with hearing health care clinicians of the highest caliber who insist on the best practice (often setting the standards for best practices) for their patients and loved ones.

❸ Does the Specialist Think Brain First?

Everybody thinks "we hear with our ears," and while that is partially correct, the process of hearing actually happens at the level of the brain. Today's hearing loss treatments are far more than a simple "amplifying" device behind your ear. The neuroscience behind modern treatments is focused on the brain, cognition, and the comorbidities of untreated hearing loss (comorbidity is defined as a disorder that co-occurs/is correlated to hearing loss). If your clinician thinks hearing first and *not* brain first in his or her treatment plan, you are missing out on many long-term lifestyle benefits. NeuroTechnology™ is aimed at restoring lost clarity, providing noise-canceling filters for noisy background situations, and soft-speech enhancers that emphasize the speech of those soft-speakers in your life.

When searching for your hearing health care provider, make sure you find a specialist that understands the significant negative impacts of untreated hearing loss on your brain. To find a local clinician who has been recognized for their commitment to thinking brain first in treatment plans, prescriptions, and protocols, you can visit the website *www.ExcellenceInAudiology.org.*

❹ Do They Include a Free Consultation at the Initial Appointment?

Most audiologists and hearing specialists offer free consultations for new patients so that you and your family can get expert advice about treatment needs, options, and timing before making this important investment.

During your first evaluation and consultation, be sure your questions are being answered, your concerns are being addressed, and you are being educated about all of your treatment options. The clinician should include a comprehensive written report during, or after, the evaluation at no charge.

❺ Does the Specialist's Office Offer Guarantees? If So, What Are They?

No matter which hearing health care provider you choose, ultimately you are not making a small investment—in both time and finances. That being said, it is important to know that your clinician is going to stand behind his or her medical treatment plan. Every Excellence in Audiology member-clinic offers multiple guarantees.

In addition to a 100% Money-Back Clarity Guarantee, be sure your specialist offers a lifetime guarantee on service and prescription programming.

Rest assured—your hearing health care is my priority. Thus, I stand by everything I've recommended in this publication and why I have chosen to lead the Excellence in Audiology movement.

❻ Is He or She Using the Latest Technology and Treatment Options Available?

Audiology today differs a great deal from years past. Computer-designed NeuroTechnology™ devices and wireless technologies dramatically increase the precision with which we restore clarity and boost hearing ability. Scientific verification of device settings, while in your ear (referred to as Real Ear Measurements) maximize the precision of NeuroTechnology™ benefits. As an added incentive, today's NeuroTechnology™ are discrete and virtually undetectable to the user and others. In fact, a new category of NeuroTechnology™, known for being invisible, can offer the most discrete, cosmetically pleasing option placed deep in your ear canal to make the entire treatment a well-kept secret!

❼ Does Your Investment Include Treatment Supplies?

Each hearing care office has its own fee schedules, and specialists often charge differently for procedures. All specialists should offer you a contract which clearly spells out the investment for you or your loved one's treatment before it begins.

❽ Does the Specialist Charge for Follow-Up and Emergency Appointments?

Each time a patient embarks on the journey of improved hearing, there is an adaptation period for the user's ears and brain to adjust. This period can take thirty to forty-five days and is individual to each patient. In addition to the complex cognitive changes that happen when restoring hearing clarity, patients will notice significant improvement in some hearing situations and perhaps not as much in some other situations. This is common in the initial process of hearing loss treatments. I believe every patient is entitled to complimentary customizations for their NeuroTechnology™ prescription.

Keep in mind, if your NeuroTechnology™ is broken or damaged due to non-compliance with care, protection, and maintenance, this may result in repair charges. As a simple rule, if you do your best to avoid breaking your NeuroTechnology™ and follow the simple guidelines that your audiology specialist shares with you, then you should have no additional costs for customizations, even if it's an "emergency."

❾ Does the Clinician Make You Feel Special and Comfortable?

When you meet with your hearing health care provider, the person you are trusting with your hearing health care, you need to be in a comfortable and welcoming environment. Each Excellence in Audiology member-clinic I work with understands the importance of hearing and the distress that can be involved with making the decision to treat one's hearing loss. The entire experience from beginning to end, including a welcoming staff, should be designed to help alleviate a person's feeling of anxiety or grief.

We believe every patient is special and must be made to feel that way every time he or she comes to one of our offices in need of hearing health care.

⑩ Does the Specialist Have a Great Reputation?

With the internet today, it is extremely easy to pull up ratings and reviews from patients. Simply go to Google and search for audiology reviews and ratings within your town. At the time of this report, my practice in Worcester, Massachusetts, and our Intermountain Audiology clinics in the west, along with Excellence in Audiology member-clinics across the country have amassed thousands of five-star reviews on Google, Facebook, and HealthyHearing.com. No other network even comes close to this number of reviews. In fact, most of our offices have other providers in their area that have either no ratings or many poor ratings.

And don't be shy about asking for references—go directly to the source! You have the right to call any audiology office and ask for a list of references, including other patients and local physicians that have volunteered to help advise patients as they first enter the (sometimes overwhelming) world of hearing loss and to help patients understand rehabilitation experiences from the first-person perspective.

QUESTION #4

How early in life should I have my hearing evaluated?

The Simple Answer

If you are over fifty, you should have your hearing evaluated.

Detailed Answer

I have tried to stress the importance of early diagnosis and treatment of hearing loss throughout this book and to each of my patients.

The American Speech Language Hearing Association, the American Academy of Audiology, and the American Medical Association have all considered the recommendation of including "hearing evaluation/screening" between the ages of fifty to sixty years young. I often use the catch phrase "Ears and Rears" as my way of getting people to remember to have their hearing checked when they turn fifty (and of course, have a colon cancer screening too!).

Similar to going to your primary care physician every year, obtaining a baseline hearing test can help to better serve you and your clinician as a guide to the medical recommendation at current or future appointments. Obtaining a baseline evaluation and discovering that you have normal hearing never hurt anyone!

Regardless of age, if you are noticing any of the symptoms of hearing loss (e.g. difficulty hearing in noisy situations, difficulty hearing the TV compared to others), if your family is suggesting you get a hearing test, or if you have ringing in your ears (defined as tinnitus), then it is time to take the first step and have your hearing evaluated and discuss treatment options.

Unfortunately, waiting too long can significantly impact the expectations and outcome of treatment, and sadly every hearing health care clinician I know has a patient they have had to tell he or she waited too long and the benefits of treatment will be minimal.

PART 2

FIXING THE RIGHT THINGS AT THE RIGHT TIME

QUESTION #5

What will happen at the initial evaluation and consultation?

Every process has a beginning, middle, and end.

The Beginning

First things first…your specialist will ask you "Why are you here to-day?" (or some variation of that "why" question). This helps to set the stage for understanding your specific hearing related issues, concerns, and experiences. This conversation is the baseline to helping your specialist understand why you "raised your hand and are seeking help." While my job title may be "audiologist," this initial line of questioning is designed to help me better understand my patient at a deeper, more emotional level. I want to know my patient's experience with hearing loss and how it impacts his/her life. How does your hearing loss impact your relationship with your grandchildren? How does hearing loss impact your relationship with your spouse? Does hearing loss get in the way of your performance at work? Some of my patients wait their entire life to go fishing with their grandchild, and now their hearing loss is robbing them of the richness of that experience and getting in the way of developing a deeper relationship. As an audiologist, it is my job to treat **_your_** hearing loss and **_you_** as a person.

The Middle

Treating hearing loss is a process steeped in science, engineering, technology, and clinical medicine. There is also an "art" to treating hearing loss, and this skill is developed with years of experience. In order to develop the right treatment plan for each patient, first there must be the proper diagnostic procedures that test every aspect of hearing.

First your clinician will observe the ear canal to make sure the canals are free of any obstructing cerumen (ear wax). This is most often followed by a procedure called tympanometry that can rule out any medical condition causing hearing loss involving the eardrum and/or the space behind it, including the middle ear bones (the "Hammer, Anvil, and Stirrup").

The Beeps!

From there, it is important to establish the degree of hearing loss (ranked from mild to profound). Using the "raise your hand when you hear the beep" may conjure memories of having your hearing screened by the school nurse, but it still serves a purpose: establishing the degree of hearing loss. If your specialist stops testing you at that point and makes a recommendation for treating your hearing loss…I advise you to run as fast as you can! The information gathered from this test, although important, is only a piece of the puzzle.

The Words!

The most important testing we will perform is designed to assess your cognitive hearing, e.g. how well do you understand words in quiet and with background noise (after all, nobody comes to the office complaining that they can't hear beeps!). This line of testing will truly help your clinician understand how well you hear, and how well you process words and conversation.

Testing a patient's ability to hear words is often referred to as "Word Discrimination Scores/Ability." First the patient is asked to repeat a list of words at a near-normal conversational volume. Individuals with normal hearing will always correctly repeat between 96-100% of the words on this test. Individuals with hearing loss will not score nearly as well. For example, many people with a mild to moderate hearing age-related hearing loss will typically score between 50-60%—thus the patient is expected to miss 40-50% of what is said to him or her on a daily basis (especially when visual and contextual cues are removed and only hearing is utilized).

The next test is a repeat, almost exactly as just described, but performed a second time at a volume and clarity setting ideal for the specific patient's hearing loss. The result of this second round of word testing is referred to as the patient's "Hearing Potential Score." Most often the patient who formerly scored between 50-60% will now score 90% and greater; thus, treatment with NeuroTechnology™ is expected to improve the patient's hearing clarity to 90% and greater on a daily basis (especially in a quiet conversational setting). The patient is fully aware that he or she performed significantly better with enhanced clarity.

I mentioned earlier that the consequences of waiting too long to treat hearing loss can be dire. In some cases when the second round of word testing is completed, the patient's "Hearing Potential Score" will sometimes only be as high as 50-60%. In these cases, the outcomes and expectations for treatment are very dim (especially when compared with the patient who scored over 90%).

The Words In Background Noise!

The #1 complaint of every patient with hearing loss, and most often the first symptom of hearing loss, is difficulty understanding speech and conversation in background noise. Thus, it is critical that the clinician understands each patient's ability to decipher speech in background noise (again, without visual or contextual cues). This test, called the Quick Speech in Noise Test (QuickSIN™), is a means to quantify a patient's difficulty understanding and following speech in background noise.

Briefly, the sentence intended to be heard and repeated by the listener is presented at a clear and audible volume to the patient. With each new sentence introduced, the level of background noise (often referred to as "cocktail party noise") is increased in increments of five decibels. The final iteration of the test is when the speech and background "babble" are presented at the same volume—significantly taxing the auditory system and its noise-reduction filters.

Individuals with normal hearing are typically capable of hearing every word at each level, and even most of the words at the final, most competitive level. In contrast, individuals with even a mild hearing loss can struggle significantly on this test when the noise is ten decibels less than the intended speech. The test is scored on a Hearing Handicap Scale and can range from normal, to mild, to moderate, to severe Hearing Handicap. A majority of patients with a mild age-related hearing loss will often score in the mild to moderate hearing handicap range, confirming his or her reported difficulty following conversation in complex listening situations.

The End

Once all the testing is complete, it is the clinician's responsibility to review all test results with the patient and with his or her loved ones. These results are personal and can help a patient better understand the difficulty he or she is dealing with on a daily basis. Understanding the results can also be just as important for family and loved ones.

Although an individual with normal hearing can only imagine what it feels like to suffer from permanent hearing loss, gaining an understanding of the degree of hearing loss, Hearing Potential Ability, and Hearing Handicap scores can help the loved ones gain perspective on what the patient is going through and how much of a strain hearing loss can be.

These test results will determine the medical treatment plan and help initiate the journey towards improved hearing clarity and cognitive health.

QUESTION #6

What if I still have questions after the initial consultation?

The initial consultation can be overwhelming for some people and for their family members—and can sometimes stretch to sixty minutes or more. In these situations, it can be difficult to ask every question, to process everything that is being said, and to understand the enormity of the diagnosis of hearing loss. Every patient of mine has my e-mail, office phone number, and I've even gone so far as to include my cell phone number on my business card. I believe in an open discussion and dialogue and that many patients, and perhaps their family members, will have questions that come up even after the appointment is over.

I always invite and encourage patients to bring family and loved ones to their appointments. Bring a spouse, bring a child, bring a grandchild—it's okay because your hearing loss impacts every one of these people.

It is important that the patient and his or her loved ones understand exactly what is happening with the patient, exactly what the degree of hearing loss is, how the disorder can impact his or her life, how it can impact his or her cognitive function, and how it can impact his or her risk of developing dementia, which often leads to loss of independence and even institutionalization. At the initial consultation, there will also be a medical recommendation presented for how to treat the hearing loss. There is no one-size-fits-all treatment plan. NeuroTechnology™ offers a wide array of options that are often dictated by the test results and patients' needs.

QUESTION #7

When is the best time to treat my hearing loss?

A.S.A.P. Hearing loss is associated with increased rates of diabetes, heart disease, kidney disease, thyroid disease, falling, and the development of dementia.

The longer you wait, the more you are depriving the brain of proper auditory stimulation, often referred to as *auditory deprivation.* Your brain is not getting the proper auditory stimulation and auditory cues that it needs to run at 100%. The brain is a very simple "Use it or Lose It" mechanism, and auditory input can help to provide the proper, constant stimulation our brains are accustomed to and designed to receive.

Hearing is not a sense to take for granted. Yet the statistics are alarming—it is estimated that only 20% of individuals with hearing loss actually seek medical treatment. Without the proper treatment of hearing loss, the brain is being asked to work on overload, constantly. I often use the analogy "living with untreated hearing loss is like asking your brain to drive sixty miles per hour in second gear."

In neuroscience, we call this "Cognitive Overload"—asking the brain to process auditory, visual, and other cues just to put together a simple sentence.

Consider this sentence:

> *Hi, Martha! How is your puppy doing? Is he eating and growing OK? I hope we can get our dogs together soon to play.*

If we filter this sentence through a typical mild age-related hearing loss with compromised clarity (e.g. difficulty with consonant discrimination), the sentence could be perceived as this:

> *i, Mara! ow i our uy oing? I e eaing and groing o? I oe e an ge our do ogeer oon o ay.*

I think you will agree that this is rather alarming. Remember earlier when we discussed patients with mild hearing loss missing 50-60% of words at near-normal conversational volume? This is what it could sound like to the patient with auditory-only cues. Of course, the brain will use visual cues, lip-reading, etc. to fill in the missing pieces—but the brain was not designed to take on that much stress and effort just to understand a simple sentence.

This cognitive overload is hypothesized to be one of the leading reasons that individuals with hearing loss can be ***FIVE TIMES*** more likely to develop dementia.

QUESTION #8

What if I am nervous about treating my hearing loss?

Undergoing treatment for any medical disorder can be overwhelming to patients and to their family members. Fortunately, today's Neuro-Technology™ has alleviated most of the worries and concerns about treating hearing loss. The technology is specifically designed to be discretely worn all day and fit comfortably in the patient's ear. With enhanced clarity features, background noise cancellation filters, and wireless connectivity, today's hearing loss treatment options are simple and sometimes even fun—you can connect your NeuroTechnology™ to all sorts of home electronics including light bulbs, coffee pots, door bells, etc.—but this is beyond the scope of this book!

QUESTION #9

Why can't we wait until next year to treat my hearing loss?

Hearing loss, for some reason, seems to be the perfect thing for patients to try and put off "until next year." Patients will try to rationalize their hearing loss: "Oh, this is normal for my age" or "Everybody mumbles." If patients don't understand the unintended consequences of waiting to treat hearing loss and the medical conditions associated with hearing loss, how can they be expected to understand the importance of starting treatment of hearing loss **today!**

Simply stated, the organ of hearing (i.e. the cochlea) has a finite amount of receptor cells—referred to as hair cells. The hair cells are akin to the rods and cones of the eye, which receive stimulation and pass along the information as a complex series of neurochemical signals to the brain. As we age, like most mammals roaming the planet, humans are genetically predetermined to suffer the effects of age-related hearing loss. This problem is becoming more prominent in our society as we live longer, more active and engaged lives.

With this progressive degenerative disorder, there is a gradual, continual loss of hair cells within the cochlea. These cells each have upwards of thirty nerve fibers responsible for relaying information to the brain to process sounds and conversation. As each cell dies with age and excessive exposure to noise (compounded by the combination of the two), the cells will die and so, too, will the attached neurons.

A recent study from Johns Hopkins found significant cerebral atrophy (AKA brain shrinkage) in the brains of individuals with hearing loss—likely the result of the progressive degenerative nature of hearing loss. The cerebral atrophy found in these individuals is reminiscent of the global cerebral atrophy observed in individuals with dementia.

Treating hearing loss early has many advantages—predicated on "Use It or (Continue to) Lose It." Treating hearing loss cannot prevent further damage caused by our genetics or prior exposure to loud noise, but it can help maintain clarity and fine resolution of speech understanding as the disorder progresses. For example, a study I worked on at Brooklyn College (CUNY) graduate school under the supervision of Dr. Shlomo Silman was attempting to understand the impact of only using one hearing aid when the patient had equal amounts of hearing loss in both ears. The results were pretty alarming.

The untreated ear's ability to perform word discrimination tasks significantly reduced compared to the treated ear. Looking back on these results, they almost seem like common sense—the brain was designed to receive input from two ears and can respond adversely if only stimulated by one. I often joke with my patients who ask, "Do I have to treat both ears?" by asking them "How many *Monopoly-men* do you know walking around with a monocle!" In all seriousness, the importance of treating hearing loss early cannot be understated. Maintaining the strength and vitality of neural connections of the ear to the brain is key to the successful treatment of hearing loss.

PART 3

FOCUSING ON A PLAN
THAT WORKS FOR YOU

Is there an ideal patient?

The ideal patient is a person who understands both the medical and personal consequences of untreated hearing loss. A person who understands that his/her hearing loss is not just about him/her, but that hearing loss impacts his/her entire family, group of friends, and community. An ideal patient is somebody who is invested in his/her life, somebody who is invested in active aging, somebody who is invested in living independently, somebody who wants to stay engaged and who wants to be a part of the conversation, somebody who wants to be a part of his/her family and who wants to be a part of their community.

The ideal patient has to accept the cost-benefit ratio when it comes to treating hearing loss; and I hope that this book has helped patients understand that it's nearly impossible to put a dollar value on improved health. I believe the ideal patient truly wants to stay involved, wants to grow, wants to remain independent, and wants to make the most of every day and every relationship that he or she has. That is an ideal patient. If you are, or know someone that fits this description, please help them begin treatment of their hearing loss as soon as possible. You are always welcome at my center or at one of the Excellence in Audiology member-clinics in your area.

I suppose on the other side of the coin is the "not ideal patient"— the person who has his wife, his kids, and his grandkids basically pushing him into the office. That's not an ideal patient, although we have helped motivate many of them to realize what they need to do for themselves and their families. This type of patient must realize the severity of their situation and they must want to make a change. As you know, "you can lead a horse to water, but you can't make it drink."

QUESTION #10

What treatment options are available to me when I'm ready to start treating my hearing loss?

I get this question often as I travel the country meeting new patients, and even from family and friends. My answer is always the same: **NeuroTechnology**™. Advances in technology specifically designed to treat the cognitive aspects of hearing loss, not just make things louder, have significantly improved patient care and patient satisfaction.

But, my next response is always "*You must see an Excellence in Audiology member-clinic to determine which form of NeuroTechnology*™ *suits you and your hearing loss best.*"

While the most important factor in determining treatment is always based on the patient's hearing profile and health care history, specific options can be based on several factors including: addressing specific patient symptoms (difficulty in certain acoustic environments, tinnitus, etc.), dexterity (can the patient manipulate an invisible hearing device?), and personal preferences (color, size, etc.,). Your hearing health care provider can help you understand which form of NeuroTechnology™, what shape and size, and which specific features can help you hear your best and keep you engaged in conversation.

QUESTION #11

What treatment options are available for the ringing in my ears (aka tinnitus)?

As a Neuroscientist and Clinical Audiologist, one of the most common questions, **and complaints**, I get from my patients is about the 'ringing' in their ears! Tinnitus (pronounced either TIH·nih·tus or tuh·NYE·tus) is defined as a sensation of sound in your ears, sometimes in your head. Each person with tinnitus has a different sound experience; for most it is described as a "ringing" sound, but many patients also report a shooshing, buzzing, or wooshing sound—similar to the sounds inside a conch shell.

It is currently estimated that nearly 50,000,000 American adults live with tinnitus. Tinnitus is experienced by approximately 80% of people living with hearing loss.

Too many people dismiss the ringing, when in fact this sound essentially represents an internal alarm alerting you that something is not as it should be. Whether the tinnitus is constant, only noticeable in a quiet room or at night, pulsating or seems to have certain triggers (i.e. exercise or caffeine), it is important that the root cause of the problem be determined and a proper treatment plan be put in place with your hearing health care specialist. In some people, the tinnitus can interfere with daily life and result in depression, anxiety and affect concentration.

What is the cause of tinnitus?

The most common cause of tinnitus is damage to the sensory organ of hearing, the cochlea (i.e. the inner ear). The cochlea is to hearing what your eyes are to vision. Within the cochlea are tiny hair-like cells, called hair cells. When these cells are damaged, the nerves that connect the hair cells to the brain (and give us the ability to hear), become permanently damaged; and often times the ringing will ensue.

How Do the Sensory Cells In My Ear Get Damaged?

The sensory cells in the ear are most vulnerable to aging. Think about it—as we get older, we tend not to see as well or see as sharply as we used to, especially in low-light environments. Unfortunately, the same process happens in our ears as we age; we tend not to hear as clearly, especially in noisy situations.

Another common cause of tinnitus is excessive noise exposure, either a single intense noise (like a shotgun blast) or long-term exposure either from work or play (e.g. musicians, concert attendees, carpenters, machinist, landscapers, etc.).

But Why Do My Ears Ring?

Tinnitus is most often the result of a "Central Gain" in neural activity that occurs when there is a loss of proper neural stimulation from the ear to the brain. More simply, when the brain is not properly stimulated in individuals with hearing loss (even a mild hearing loss), the brain will increase activity to make up for the missing input.

This "Central Gain" is neurologically analogous to "Phantom Limb" phenomenon studied in neuroscience. In cases where damage occurs to the peripheral nervous system—such as when a solider loses a limb in battle—the central nervous system (aka the brain) will undergo adaptive changes that can often result in the perception of pain. Our ear's perception of pain is the ringing.

Treatment For Your Tinnitus

Unfortunately, too many patients have said to me, "I have tinnitus, and I've been told there is nothing that I can do about it." I emphatically say to each of these patients—that is not true! Is there a cure for tinnitus? No. Are there proven FDA-approved treatment options available to reduce, and in some cases, eliminate, the ringing? YES!

The single most effective treatment option available for patients suffering with tinnitus is NeuroTechnology™. The FDA (Food and Drug Administration) has approved treatment for individuals with tinnitus by providing the brain with restored proper stimulation. And while most people with tinnitus also suffer with hearing loss, that is not always the case. Fortunately, newly available NeuroTechnology™ has been designed for people with hearing loss and for individuals with (so called) "normal" hearing. Many studies show that patients who use the tinnitus support technology note a significant reduction in their daily tinnitus experience—with some even reporting that "the ringing is gone all day."

QUESTION #12

What if I have "total hearing loss" in one of my ears? (And what is a CROS System?)

As a general rule of thumb, hearing ability in the two ears should be near equal to each other. After all, your ears are the same age. If you have a history of noise exposure it was likely the same in both ears, and if you were prescribed a medicine with a side-effect that could impact hearing, it would impact both ears similarly.

But, in some patients, hearing in one ear will diverge from the other. This can result from a host of otologic issues, including viral infection of the ear, physical trauma to the ear, and of unknown origin (medically diagnosed as "idiopathic hearing loss," which is my favorite medical diagnosis because the root meaning of the phrase "idiopathic" is that the clinicians are idiots and don't know what happened! Ha! I don't say that to disparage any clinicians—it's just sometimes we can't figure out why the patient has worse hearing in one ear).

The separation of hearing levels between the two ears can sometimes be dramatic or even complete. Unfortunately, some patients have a "dead ear" (medically defined as anacusis) with normal hearing in the other ear. In other patients, there is an "asymmetric hearing loss" which implies hearing loss in one ear and even worse hearing in the other ear.

The brain was designed to hear with two ears, and it will function best with equal hearing in both ears. Binaural (two-ear) hearing has significant benefits that include increased sound localization ability (e.g. figuring out where sound is coming from in the room) and enhanced perception of speech in noisy situations. These characteristics of binaural hearing are often referred to as the "Binaural Advantage." If you know somebody with "lopsided" hearing loss, you will notice that she always strategizes to improve the listening environment by having the speaker(s) on her better hearing side.

While the course of treatment for individuals with significantly poorer hearing in one ear is different than the patient with symmetrical hearing loss, NeuroTechnology™ can be used to significantly enhance hearing and understanding in all listening situations.

Briefly, the most common NeuroTechnology™ used in these cases is referred to as a CROS System. CROS (Contralateral Routing of Signal) will take sound from the "dead" / worse side and route it over to the better side (even if there is some hearing loss in the "better" side). Using this technology allows the patient to access sound on the (otherwise) muted side of the body. While this patient may never perform as well as an individual treating equal levels of hearing loss in both ears, restoring perception of sound from the muted side of the body can offer significant relief in almost all listening situations.

QUESTION #13

Do they still make traditional hearing aids?

Yes, traditional hearing aids are still made. Mostly this traditional technology has been relabeled and is now masquerading as "new" over-the-counter (OTC) technology or personal sound amplification devices (PSAPs). Unfortunately, because the words "hearing aid" are very general and very common, it can be quite confusing for the patient. As I explain to my patients nearly every day:

"Your father (or grandfather) wore traditional hearing aids (and he probably hated them). This older technology was intended to make sounds louder regardless of location in the room, regardless of the volume of the incoming sounds, and regardless of what the patient did or didn't actually want to hear."

As an audiologist seeing patients early on in my career, I was very disappointed by the limitations of the traditional hearing aid technology (and often embarrassed about having to relay the cost of the device— knowing the benefit would be limited, thereby limiting the patient's ability to remain socially engaged). This high level of patient dissatisfaction played a role in my decision to "take a break" from clinical audiology for nearly six years and pursue my studies in neuroscience.

QUESTION #14

So, what's the deal with new hearing aids and NeuroTechnology™?

(Most) new "hearing aids" are NeuroTechnology™.

To continue my answer from the last question: when I decided to come back to audiology as a clinical fellow at the Brigham and Women's Hospital in Boston and then as clinical professor at Northeastern University, I was instantly relieved at the giant leaps and bounds hearing aids had made towards improving listening experience for the patient (and thus increasing patient satisfaction). Around this time, the average patient satisfaction rating for traditional hearing aid experience was hovering around 70% to75% (as measured by the MarkeTrak survey).

If you now fast-forward another ten years to present time, the most recent MarkeTrack survey examining patient satisfaction with hearing loss treatment has shown an **improvement to 91%!** I believe this number speaks for itself.

Treatment of hearing loss with traditional hearing aids is (thankfully) beginning to be phased out and replaced with NeuroTechnology™ designed to enhance hearing in all listening situations, enhance clarity of speech details, automatically provide an increased boost of volume for soft speakers, stimulate the brain, and increase cognitive function.

QUESTION #15

What in the heck is an invisible hearing aid?

I saved my favorite treatment topic for last…*invisible hearing aids*. Like Wonder Woman's invisible jet plane—you can't see it, but it kicks butt! I get questions about this all the time from patients: "What is an invisible hearing aid?" and "Will my friends be able to see it?"

When treating hearing loss with NeuroTechnology™, I have two principles that I always follow:

1. Use the right NeuroTechnology™ to treat the patient's hearing loss and improve cognitive health.

2. Respect the patient's desire for NeuroTechnology™ that is physically and aesthetically comfortable for them.

BUT… Principle #2 can _never_ override Principle #1.

As a general rule of thumb in the tech world, the size of technology decreases over time. NeuroTechnology™ uses smaller, more powerful digital technology and processing to automatically adapt to the user's surroundings. I have always believed that treating hearing loss should require minimal effort from the patient. The hearing-impaired person needs to start using NeuroTechnology™ when he or she wakes up in the morning and then simply remove it before falling asleep—and do *nothing* in between! NeuroTechnology™ has ushered in the age of *effortless* hearing loss treatment.

Advances in design and technology allow for the user to be hands free—no more buttons for environment (i.e. push the button twice when in a noisy restaurant, push three times when in the gym, push the button four times when on the phone, etc.) and no more spin-wheels to adjust the volume up and down. Innovations in NeuroTechnology™ allow for automatic adaptation to dynamic environmental listening situations (e.g. listening to speech as you go from a quiet room to a noisy room), and it can automatically adapt to incoming volume to maintain the normal fluctuations in the volume of voices and background noise. The most advanced feature of NeuroTechnology™ is noise-cancellation that delivers increased access to <u>clear</u> speech in noisy listening situations (more on this in the bonus question!).

While NeuroTechnology™ is the circuitry inside the device, the device can come in different shapes and sizes to best fit your hearing loss and your ear.

NeuroTechnology™ Options for Treating Hearing Loss

Invisible Treatment Options

Once placed in your ear, this technology is hassle-free—you may even forget you're wearing the device! And that's the point. Hearing loss shouldn't hold you back, and neither should your hearing solution. Features in today's invisible technology options include:

- An invisible and custom fit
- A deep fit inside your ear canal and personal customization to you for all-day comfort
- Easy adaptation to new sounds with automatic volume control and adaptation to the listening environment
- Wireless streaming to your smartphone to keep you connected to your TV, music, and other media

- Sound comfort technology designed to provide distortion-free listening comfort for loud sounds while ensuring ultimate clarity

Invisible technology is seated comfortably in the ear canal for all day comfort and maximum discreteness.

Mini "Receiver in the Ear" Options

Groundbreaking NeuroTechnology™ is fast and precise enough to analyze and follow the dynamics of the entire auditory environment and differentiate between speech and background noise. Briefly (and without getting too lost in technical details), NeuroTechnology™ is capable of sampling sounds in the environment 100 times per second to make a decision on how to optimally perform and restore clarity; whereas traditional hearing aids were barely capable of analyzing the sound environment and capped out at a sampling rate of less that five times per second.

Advances in miniaturization of technology have led to the breakthrough of new NeuroTechnology™ found to support brain function, including working memory, selective attention, and processing speed (see Bibliography section for report from Dr. Desjardin, University of Texas, El Paso). These new devices have three features designed specifically to maintain the brain's innate ability to hear in all different listening situations:

- **Clear Hearing in Background Noise.** By separating important speech from background noise by as much as 10 decibels, this new technology provides 30% better speech understanding and clarity in noise*.

- **Enhanced Clarity = Enhanced Memory Recall.** Individuals with hearing loss can have difficulty with working memory, thought to be the result of distorted auditory input to the brain. NeuroTechnology™ can provide 20% more capacity to recall and remember words* by increasing the clarity of the signal being processed by the brain.

- **Reduced Mental Effort.** Many patients describe hearing loss as being "exhausting." Normal hearing is relatively effortless in most listening situations. But to an individual with hearing loss, even a simple conversation at work with a colleague or while out fishing with the grandchildren can require significant effort and use of all available mental resources, including lip-reading. NeuroTechnology™ can offer the hearing-impaired user relief by reducing the "cognitive load" (e.g. mental effort) by 20%*; making the conversation significantly easier to follow in all situations.

Compared to traditional hearing aids

Other features include:

- Hands-free wireless surround sound hearing on the phone.

- Low-battery reminders. Devices can remind you by ear, phone, text, or email that your batteries (or your spouse's batteries) are low.

- Wireless compatibility with any TV to enhance the clarity of the signal.

- Control of your internet connected devices at home, including the thermostat, lights, and even certain cooking appliances.

Let's join in with all current NeuroTechnology™ users and celebrate!

Gone are the days of clunky "beige banana" hearing aids!

PART 4

FINANCING YOUR HEARING LOSS TREATMENT WITHOUT BREAKING THE BANK

QUESTION #16

How much will my "new ears" cost me?

Answer: It depends.

Throughout this book I have alluded to NeuroTechnology™ treatment options as the "gold standard" of treating hearing loss. Specific recommendations will rely on a number of factors (e.g. degree of hearing loss, symptoms, amount of time living with untreated hearing loss, etc.). However, with that said, I have over twenty years of horror stories of patients trying to *"save a buck."* I know patients who have thrown away $30, $300, even as much as $3,000 on a "sound machine in their ear" that amplifies volume. Some have tried traditional hearing aids that only make sounds louder; some have tried over-the-counter (OTC) devices; some have tried Personal Sound Amplifiers (PSAPs); some have even tried "mail-order" hearing aids. Regardless, each time the patient comes in professing his *mea culpa* and seeking forgiveness. I take no issue with patients trying to save money and make good economic decisions, but even with health care…you get what you pay for.

Treating the progressive degenerative nature of age-related hearing loss is no different than treating other major medical disorders as you age.

As an example, imagine yourself, or a loved one, in a situation where hip-replacement surgery is required. Could you imagine your surgeon asking the following question?

> *"Would you like me to replace your hip and restore 30%, 70%, or maximum percent mobility?"*

Here is another example, imagine saying to your heart surgeon, after he/she lets you know that you are required to undergo triple by-pass and heart valve replacement:

> *"Doc, if you don't mind, I'm going to shop on Amazon for a replacement valve to try and save a few bucks...even if it doesn't pump the adequate amount of blood to keep my body oxygenated and healthy."*

While both of these scenarios may seem far-fetched and ridiculous, unfortunately the retail aspect of hearing health care has "poisoned the well" for too many people living with hearing loss and has made treating hearing loss a very confusing, onerous process for the patient.

We trust all of our health care providers to use their knowledge and experience to provide us with the best, most medically sound treatment recommendation, ***regardless of price***. You should expect the same from your doctor of audiology. If your clinician is reputable (e.g. is referred to by local physicians, has many five-star reviews on Google, has readily available current patient liaisons to speak with, etc.), is an Excellence in Audiology member-clinic, and has longevity in the community, then you can rest assured that their pricing structure is standard and that the only variable is the cost of technology (pre-set by the technology manufacturer).

NeuroTechnology™ is the #1 most effective, FDA (Food and Drug Administration) approved treatment for hearing loss and has the highest recorded level of patient satisfaction.

QUESTION #17

What is the cost of <u>not</u> treating my hearing loss?

Answer: Possibly a lot more than you think!

Throughout this book we have discussed the positive impact of treating hearing loss and the dire consequences of not treating hearing loss. It is difficult to assign a true monetary value to both of these scenarios, but I will give it my best shot!

Here are two examples.

1. **Hearing loss can increase the risk of developing dementia by 200-500%.** Treating hearing loss is reported as the single most effective modifiable factor to preventing dementia. Given these two medical research findings, it is not unreasonable to calculate the cost of treating a patient with dementia that could have possibly been avoided by treating his or her hearing loss at an earlier age. Statistics show that the average family will spend approximately $57,000.00 per year to cover health care costs and manage the care of a loved one with dementia.

2. **Hearing loss increases the risk of falls in seniors.** Treating hearing loss can significantly reduce the risk of falling. Again, given these two medical research findings, it is not unreasonable to calculate the cost of treating a patient who falls and compare it to the cost of treating hearing loss. Falling over the age of sixty-five is the #1 cause of injury related deaths. And once a person falls, he or she is two times more likely to fall again. The Center for Disease Control and Prevention (CDC) estimates that the average medical cost associated with a fall that results in hospitalization is over $30,000.00 (and the cost of treatment increases with age).

In addition to dementia and falls, co-morbidity of hearing loss (i.e. other diseases that are correlated with hearing loss) extends to diabetes, coronary disease, thyroid disease, and others.

QUESTION #18

How do I pay for treatment and what is TreatmentFi™?

"Patients must be provided affordable treatment options when investing in the medical treatment of hearing loss." —Dr. Keith N. Darrow

Like any major medical procedure, the treatment of hearing loss and associated cognitive needs can be expensive, and much of it will *not* covered by your insurance. Unfortunately, price is the most common reason that patients reject the medical treatment of hearing loss. And perhaps an additional problem is that expensive traditional hearing aids never really worked—thus there was little value in paying such a high price. But that has all changed. NeuroTechnology™ is designed to treat the cognitive aspects of hearing loss, and with TreatmentFi™, treatment is now affordable and designed for patients to begin treatment on day one.

For too long I have worked with too many patients who were eager to start treatment of their hearing loss only to be held back by the cost. This motivated me to go back to the drawing board and re-think how we could make hearing health care affordable. I'm so proud that after years of many sleepless nights and way too much time dealing with lawyers and bankers, **we now offer a program that provides access to affordable hearing health care—without compromise.** In the past, if a patient wanted to save a few bucks, they had to even further reduce the effectiveness of traditional hearing aids, but this is no longer an issue for our patients.

TreatmentFi™ has been approved by all 50 state attorney generals for use as an affordable means of treating hearing loss. Each Excellence in Audiology member-clinic offers this new TreatmentFi™ program to their patients. In addition to removing the barrier for my new patients to invest in proper hearing health care, this program also tackles another major issue: patients who have traditional hearing aids but are worried about the cost of upgrading treatment with NeuroTechnology™. This is why I have devised TreatmentFi™ to include no-cost changes to technology every 3 1/2 to 4 years based on changes to the patient's hearing and cognitive needs.

The TreatmentFi™ program at Excellence In Audiology member-clinics is all-inclusive and ensures that each patient always has what is best to treat his or her hearing loss and cognitive needs. With TreatmentFi™, the leader in financing hearing health treatment, our patients have access to low-cost monthly treatment plans that provide significant benefits, including full warranty coverage on treatment technology (including loss, damage, and repair coverage for life); complete access to supplies, batteries, and service appointments; and most importantly, *no-cost automatic upgrades* on new treatment technology. The fact of the matter is that not only will a patient's hearing and cognitive needs change over time, but technology will also improve. With TreatmentFi™, treating patients is the top priority!

The benefits of treating your hearing loss with the exclusive TreatmentFi™ process are unlike any other treatment plans available to patients. Each patient that begins treatment of their hearing loss can expect the following benefits:

- A pair of adaptive NeuroTechnology™ is designed to address the cognitive aspects of hearing loss

- Lifetime hearing loss coverage with affordable fixed monthly treatment plan costs

- Lifetime warranty (including a one-time loss)

- Automatic technology upgrades every 48 months (or less)

- Access to discounted technology accessories including rechargeable batteries, smartphone, and TV adapter
- All office visits included
- Hearing technology supplies included (batteries, cleaning accessories, etc.)

The standard cost of the TreatmentFi™ can be customized depending on your hearing and cognitive needs, insurance benefits, and financial situation. Your treatment team will always develop a plan that is right for you!

The medical treatment of hearing loss is associated with a number of physical and cognitive benefits including improvements in quality of life, enhancements in cognitive function, memory recall and attention, and reducing the risk of developing dementia. Additionally, recent reports indicate that the treatment of hearing loss may even slow the *progression* of dementia. Our obligation to our patients is to make treatment accessible, and TreatmentFi™ helps more people make the right decision to treat their hearing loss today.

And don't forget—there are **no hidden costs** in this program. You pay one low monthly fee. Period.

How to Offset the Costs

Use of the TreatmentFi™ program can be customized to meet each patient's needs. Some of the ways that many of my patients cover the low monthly cost is by using their Flexible Spending Account (FSA), using their tax returns, and even writing off the cost of treatment as a medical expense benefit on their tax returns. (Warning: I am not an accountant—and I don't even play one on TV—so always ask your accountant how to best proceed with all tax matters.)

How to use Flexible Spending and eliminate the headache of using it!

Just to make sure we are all on the same page, Flex Spending is accessible through your work benefit package, and it allows you to set aside a certain amount of money per year—TAX-FREE!—to be used towards medical expenses. NeuroTechnology™ and the medical treatment of hearing loss is a medical expense.

Step 1—Sign Up Early!

Perhaps you already follow the "5 P's to Success"—Proper Planning Prevents Poor Performance! But in case you don't, this is one thing you want to plan early for so you can maximize the benefit. Many employees set higher limits than you think on the amount of Flexible Spending dollars you can contribute and access.

I have seen employees with as much as $2,500, and some with even $5,000 in Flex-Spending dollars available to them. Failure to sign up early could cost you more in out-of-pocket medical expenses, especially if your plan is not up and ready before you or a loved one needs to treat his or her hearing loss. If you have a new plan, work with your human resource contact to sign up early for next year in order to maximize your savings.

Step 2—Notify Your Employer of Family Status Changes.

Different employers have different sign-up deadlines for the Flexible Spending plans, but typically at the beginning of the year your employer asks how much money you want to contribute for the year.

The problem with making annual decisions about health care coverage is obvious—life happens and sometimes it's nearly impossible to plan that far ahead! You may apply for a family status change for events such as marriage, birth, divorce, or loss of a spouse's insurance. These are opportunities to add more coverage for hearing loss treatment expenses.

Step 3—Choose Wisely!

Give some thought to calculating how much money to contribute to your flexible plan at work this year—and every year. If you are considering hearing loss treatment for you or a family member, visit your local Excellence In Audiology member-clinic to learn about Treatment-Fi™ during initial consultation.

Your patient care coordinator can help you plan exactly how much money you should contribute to help reduce your out-of-pocket costs when it is time to pay for and receive your NeuroTechnology™.

Step 4—Use It or Lose It.

Here's something you may not know—and frankly, it's something which has always puzzled me! If you put more money into your Flex Spending Account than you need or use, by law, you lose the money! Yikes!

You do have three months after the end of the calendar year to submit claims for eligible medical expenses from the previous calendar year. But any money left in your account following this three-month period is forfeited.

QUESTION #19

Does my insurance cover the cost of NeuroTechnology™?

This is a loaded question—and one that I can only answer in general terms because health insurance coverage is a complex ever-changing set of rules, regulations, and specifics that make it impossible to make a blanket statement regarding *your* coverage.

After twenty years of patient care and working with nearly every flavor of insurance coverage, these are my two take-away messages:

1. Nearly every insurance plan, including Medicare, will cover the cost of the comprehensive hearing evaluation.

2. Many patients have some coverage for the cost of treatment (e.g. NeuroTechnology™).

I acknowledge that "nearly every" and "many" are vague terms, but this is the world of insurance we currently live in. I have worked with patients that have $100 of coverage and some with $10,000 in coverage (not that it should ever cost you that much!).

TIP: Do not be afraid to pick up the phone and ask your insurance company point blank: **"Do you cover the cost of treating hearing loss?"** Also, don't be afraid to call back and ask again (you would be shocked how many times our office has called insurance companies seeking this answer only to get a different answer each time we call!). At my office, our Patient Care Coordinators will take the guess work out of the patient's hands and will work directly with the insurance company, and fight with them when needed, to maximize the patient's benefits and coverage.

BONUS SECTION

TREATING HEARING LOSS & YOUR OVERALL HEALTH

QUESTION #20

What is the research behind the relationship of hearing loss and dementia?

Age-Related Hearing Loss is a progressive and degenerative disorder resulting from the loss of receptor cells (i.e. the hair cells) in the ear. Consequently, there is a significant reduction of the quantity and quality of neural connections from the ear to the brain. This slow-onset disorder can have a significant impact on several key brain areas, including the memory, hearing, speech and language portions of cognitive function. Several key research studies have pointed to the potential links of hearing loss and dementia, including the groundbreaking work from Dr. Lin and his colleagues at Johns Hopkins Medical Center that indicate **hearing loss can increase the risk of Dementia by 200-500%.**

Summary data of relationship of hearing loss and increased risk of developing dementia.

The initial report first published in 2011 by scientists at Johns Hopkins Medical Center and the National Institute on Aging found that individuals with hearing loss (when compared to participants with normal hearing) are at a significantly higher risk of developing dementia as they age. The relationship of hearing loss and increased risk was rather simple: the more hearing loss they had, the higher the likelihood of developing the memory-robbing disease. "A lot of people ignore hearing loss because it's such a slow and insidious process as we age," Dr. Frank Lin (of Johns Hopkins Medical Center) says. "Even if people feel as if they are not affected, we're showing that it may well be a more serious problem."

Three risk factors associated with hearing loss and dementia include Social Isolation, Cerebral Atrophy and Cognitive Overload.

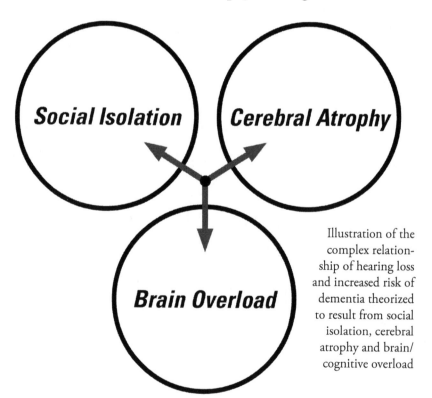

Illustration of the complex relationship of hearing loss and increased risk of dementia theorized to result from social isolation, cerebral atrophy and brain/cognitive overload

1. Social Isolation

The Impact of reduced social and physical activity. Withdrawal from social situations is common in individuals with hearing loss. Many studies cite feelings of embarrassment, fear of making mistakes in conversations, and feeling like you are not part of the conversation as the common rational for individuals with hearing impairment to separate themselves from family, friends and community. This retreat from social activity has even been found in individuals with a mild degree of hearing loss. In addition, individuals with hearing loss are less likely to engage in physical activity. Both increased social isolation and reduced physical activity are strong risk factors for the development of Dementia.

> *Blindness Separates You from Things,*
> *Deafness Separates You from People.*
> *— Helen Keller*

Active Aging: How to Reduce Social Isolation

Active Aging—the process of optimizing opportunities for better health, continuing development of knowledge, and increased security in order to maximize quality of life as you age. The word "active" is used to describe a person's involvement with social, physical, economic, spiritual and civic affairs. We all share the same goal to maintain autonomy and independence as we age, and thus we must rely on preserving the tenants of interdependence (socialization and reliance on family and loved ones) and intergenerational solidarity (maintaining companionship with age-matched peers) to insure active aging.

Both Social Isolation and Depression are risk factors for the development of dementia, and both increase as we age. Being a lifelong learner and staying active is important to maintain a healthy, active brain, and can also reduce your risk of cognitive decline and dementia. Some studies have shown that social activities, larger social networks, and a history of social contact are associated with better cognitive function and reduced risk for cognitive decline.

Tips for Active Aging include:

- Sharing a meal with family and friends 3–5 times per week
- Committing to an aerobics/exercise regiment
- Learning a new hobby each year
- Playing an instrument (or learning a new instrument)
- If you love to read…keep reading (and try to mix up the topics!)
- If you don't read much—try to read a book every other month
- Participating in classes at your local senior center
- Volunteering at a local hospital, shelter, etc.
- Going back to school. Many local state Universities offer free tuition to people over 65!

2. Cerebral Atrophy (AKA Brain Shrinkage)

The association of a shrinking brain, resulting from the loss of neurons, with dementia has been long documented. Even people with MCI (Mild Cognitive Impairment) show signs of cerebral atrophy. In recent years, scientific studies using advanced brain imaging techniques (including fMRI - Functional Magnetic Resonance Imaging) have demonstrated that hearing impairment is associated with accelerated brain atrophy in both the overall brain, as well as even more advanced reductions in volume associated with the memory, hearing, speech and language portions of the brain.

Individuals with hearing loss can experience significant cerebral atrophy. The most significant reduction in cerebral volume occurs in areas involved in memory, hearing, speech and language.

Brain With Hearing Loss   **Brain With Normal Hearing**

Schematic representing the potential cerebral atrophy in an individual with age-related hearing loss.

3. Cognitive Overload (i.e. Working Your Brain Too Hard to Hear)

Hearing loss is not normal, and neither is the excessive strain that it can put on your brain. If you or somebody you love is experiencing hearing loss, you can observe this strain by watching the amount of effort required to follow a conversation. Patients will often joke and say "I need to put my glasses on so I can hear you better." Requiring these extra visual and lip-reading cues may seem a natural way to fill in the missing speech details, but long term these coping mechanisms may have harmful effects on cognitive function.

With hearing loss, the brain is constantly on "overload" trying to fill in the missing pieces, and follow the conversation. I often describe to my patients the taxing effect of hearing loss on brain function by describing the mental effort required to hear "is like driving 60 miles per hour in only second gear."

Increased cognitive load is considered a risk factor for developing dementia. Cognitive load, as measured by pupillometry (i.e. the size of the pupils indicates the amount of mental effort), can quantify how hard your brain is working to follow a conversation. Recent studies have found that individuals who treat their hearing loss do not work as hard to listen (i.e. have a reduced cognitive load) and have as much as a 20% increase in memory recall when following a conversation, even in noisy environments.

QUESTION #21

Can I reduce my increased risk of developing dementia by treating my hearing loss?

As I discuss the relationship of hearing loss and dementia with my patients, each seems to have the same follow up question for me: *"Doc, if I treat my hearing loss, can I prevent or reduce my risk of developing dementia?"*

Thankfully, the data appears to be trending towards a resounding "*Yes!*" Recent reports have found a significant positive impact of treating hearing loss on cognitive health.

Treating Hearing Loss and the Impact on Cognitive Function

In a recent study investigating the relationship of treating hearing loss and cognitive function, it was found that current hearing loss treatments can improve brain function in people with hearing loss. It is understood that hearing loss, if left untreated, can lead to emotional and social consequences, reduced job performance, and diminished quality of life. Recently, studies have even shown that untreated hearing loss can interfere with cognitive abilities because so much mental effort is diverted toward understanding speech (i.e. cognitive overload).

The research was aimed at measuring core cognitive functions in subjects in their 50's and 60's beginning hearing loss treatment for the first time. After only two weeks of treatment, cognitive testing began to reveal a significant increase in scores for recalling words in working memory and selective attention tests, and that the processing speed for which participants selected the correct response was significantly faster. In summary: after only a couple of weeks, participants exhibited significant improvement in their cognitive function.

Treating Hearing Loss and the Impact on Risk of Developing Dementia

Since 2011, multiple long-term studies have provided strong evidence that treating hearing loss may eliminate the increased risk of developing dementia. **Dr. Lalwani at Columbia University noted that treating hearing loss...**

> *may offer a simple, yet important, way to prevent or slow the development of dementia by keeping adults with hearing loss engaged in conversation and communication.*

Perhaps the most definitive report comes from the Lancet Commission, which presented a new life-course model documenting potentially modifiable risk factors for dementia. The Commission's report suggests that treating hearing loss is the **single most effective modifiable factor to preventing dementia.** Other modifiable factors include reducing depression, increasing physical activity and reducing social isolation – each of which is positively impacted by treating hearing loss.

QUESTION #22

Can I really expect to be more socially active and engaged once I start treating my hearing loss?

Yes. Throughout this book, I have been providing countless examples of how treating hearing loss can profoundly impact a patient's life and mental health. Frankly, connecting the dots of treating hearing loss to improvements in overall health and personal independence is simple.

If you ask your primary care physician "Doc, what do I need to do to be healthier?", the answer is guaranteed to include reduce stress, increase physical activity, stay socially active and engaged, lose weight, and eat healthy. Treating your hearing loss can help you achieve most of these goals. And achieving these goals is the key to healthy active aging.

There are countless medical studies that find that people who do not treat hearing loss suffer from increased rates of depression, decreased socialization, and decreased physical activity. As an example, the National Council on Aging reported that individuals who do *not* treat hearing loss suffer from depression, anxiety, and decreased social activity. In contrast, individuals who proactively treat their hearing loss find improvements in relationships with family members (spouse, children, grandchildren, etc.), increased self-esteem, and improvements in overall quality of life.

Connecting the Dots of Treating Hearing Loss and Improving Your Life

- Treating hearing loss can increase physical activity, reduce stress and anxiety, help with losing weight, and ultimately mean living a healthier and more independent lifestyle.

- Treating hearing loss can increase clarity of speech and the ability to follow conversation in background noise, increase socialization, help reduce the risk of depression, and ultimately mean living a healthier and more independent lifestyle.

- Treating hearing loss can increase auditory and environmental awareness, decrease the risk of falls, and ultimately mean living a healthier and more independent lifestyle.

- Treating hearing loss can increase cognitive function, can reduce the increased risk of developing dementia, and ultimately mean living a healthier and more independent lifestyle.

Hearing loss can be isolating for so many people for a multitude of reasons. **But it doesn't have to be.** If you've made it this far through the book, you have come to understand the importance of treating hearing loss and taking care of your brain—and how these two are connected.

I wish you luck and happiness as you embark on the journey of treating hearing loss, restoring clarity, increasing independence, and keeping a healthy and fit brain!

EPILOGUE

You Had Questions and I hope I've Provided Answers

S O, THERE YOU HAVE IT! Twenty-two of my patients' most popular questions answered (for your convenience I've included a handy FAQ directly after this epilogue that summarizes most, if not all, of the questions we've just covered. Consider it a handy "quick reference" of sorts).

The fact is no book can ever answer EVERY question for every patient. Every case is unique, just as every patient with hearing loss that I treat is different. What I've tried to do is provide you with the basics and, hopefully, the confidence you'll need to ask further questions of your own hearing care specialist when the time comes.

This is your hearing, your brain, and your overall health we are talking about here; never be afraid to insist on being heard and having your questions answered by your clinician. Now that you're armed with the answers for today's most frequently asked audiology questions, you can finally make the right decision for you or a loved one when embarking on the journey of medical treatment for hearing loss.

When you are ready to take the next step to improve your life, your cognitive function, and your hearing health, please visit:

www.AZBalanceAndHearing.com
or call **1(520) 263-8099**
to Schedule a Consultation

FAQS

A RESOURCE GUIDE OF FREQUENTLY ASKED QUESTIONS & TERMINOLOGY

What might happen if I wait to treat my hearing loss?

Even mild hearing loss can be a major problem for a number of reasons. Hearing loss can increase the risk of developing dementia and is correlated with several other major diseases including diabetes, coronary disease, and kidney disease. Early treatment also improves the treatment prognosis and expected outcomes.

Who are some famous people who've invested in treating their hearing loss with technology?

The list is quite long! A (much) abbreviated list includes presidents Reagan, Clinton, and George H.W. Bush, and other celebrities and famous athletes including Huey Lewis, Lou Ferrigno, William Shatner, Pete Townshend, Whoopi Goldberg, Derrick Coleman, Congressman Jim Ryun, Phil Collins, and Brian Kerwin.

Will I be able to afford NeuroTechnology™?

Yes. TreatmentFi™ provides the highest level of hearing health care to meet your hearing loss and cognitive needs, all at an affordable, set, low, monthly price!

Will being fit with NeuroTechnology™ be painful or obvious to others?

No and no. Advances in miniaturization of technology have helped develop the most light-weight, discrete, and sometimes completely invisible technology ever used to treat hearing loss.

Will I have to miss work or other social activities once fit with NeuroTechnology™?

The initial comprehensive evaluation and treatment procedures will take between one to one and a half hours. Follow-up visits after that will only take between fifteen to thirty minutes. Patients walk out of the office after the first appointment and go about their lives…only now they can hear *MUCH* better!

Is it really such a big deal if I don't treat my hearing loss?

Yes. Too many people believe that their hearing loss is "normal for their age." There is no such thing as "normal" or "age-corrected" hearing loss. Hearing loss is a progressive degenerative disorder that will continue to negatively impact your life and cognition the longer it goes untreated.

What are some of the warning signs that I may have hearing loss?

Early symptoms of hearing loss include difficulty following conversation in background noise, experiencing tinnitus (ringing in the ears), having to turn up the TV louder than others need it, asking people to repeat often, finding yourself needing to read lips to hear better, difficulty understanding on the phone, and your family bugging you about getting help.

What kind of side-effects can result from NOT treating my hearing loss?

Untreated hearing loss is implicated in increased risk of falls, development of dementia, diabetes, coronary disease, depression, as well as increased stress and reduced physical activity.

Why should I choose a specialist to treat my hearing loss?

Hearing loss is a major medical condition and has been listed as the **third most common** medical disorder impacting seniors. Unfortunately, loopholes in many state and federal laws allow for traditional hearing aids to be sold in retail establishments, including some of the big-box discount stores. These traditional hearing aids are most often older models and are only designed to amplify sound.

NeuroTechnology™, designed to treat the cognitive aspects of hearing loss, is the "gold-standard" and considered "best practices" by audiologists and board-certified specialists in private practice audiology clinics.

How do I know if my hearing care provider is a Doctor of Audiology?

This is typically pretty easy to figure out by searching the internet or even calling the office. I've never been bothered by a patient calling to confirm my credentials prior to his or her arrival—in fact, I believe this shows a proper amount of due diligence on the part of the patient and a true investment in his or her hearing health care. Most states will also provide a list or search tool online to find licensed and certified providers.

What is a Patient Care Coordinator?

During your initial consultation(s), you will usually be assigned a patient contact person—we call this person a Patient Care Coordinator in our office—with whom to schedule appointments, confer with for rescheduling, and, of course, help you get answers to any and all questions you may have at any point in the process.

Why are follow-up visits important?

These are wonderful opportunities to ask questions you may have missed the first time, get further details from your specialist, and bring a family member to learn about your diagnosis and treatment plan.

Why is early treatment so important?

Since we recommend adults fifty and older to have a comprehensive hearing evaluation, we have coined the term "Ears and Rears"! This is meant to remind people to add hearing to their list of medical appointments once they turn fifty. At fifty, if the patient is found to have hearing loss, it is critical to start treatment early to avoid some of the devastating consequences of untreated hearing loss. Alternatively, if the patient has normal hearing, a baseline will be established and used for comparison at follow-up appointments.

What if I don't believe in early treatment of age-related hearing loss?

Unfortunately, for many patients it takes nearly seven years for them to admit they have hearing loss (or to succumb to pressure from family members) and start treatment. By this time, the hearing loss will typically be at a moderate degree or beyond and, in some cases, treatment outcomes can be negatively impacted. To assure a positive prognosis and improved treatment outcomes, hearing loss must be caught early and treated early to maintain positive connections to the brain. *"Catch it early and treat it early!"*

What is sensorineural hearing loss?

Sensorineural hearing loss (SNHL) is a hearing impairment that results from damage to, or dysfunction of, the inner ear (cochlear) and/or the auditory nervous system. Age-related hearing loss is a form of sensorineural hearing loss.

What is a conductive hearing loss?

Conductive hearing loss (CHL) is a hearing impairment that results from damage to, or dysfunction of, the outer ear (pinna and ear canal) and/or the middle ear (the eardrum or ossicles—hammer, anvil and stirrup). In some cases of CHL, surgical intervention can help restore hearing function.

What is a processing disorder?

Hearing loss is often defined in terms of the amount of lost volume that results from either a SNHL or a CHL. However, many patients, even those with normal hearing levels, can have a processing disorder that will limit their ability to understand and follow speech in background noise. The noise cancellation feature in NeuroTechnology™ provides significant benefit by reducing background noise and enhancing speech—even for those with normal hearing.

Should I bring a family member with me to my appointment(s)?

I answer this with a decisive *YES*. Your hearing loss not only impacts you but also everybody around you. I have always encouraged every patient to bring a spouse or a loved one to every appointment so he or she can help me, and the patient, better understand the daily impact of hearing loss on everybody's life.

What is NeuroTechnology™?

In recent years, traditional hearing aids, which simply make sounds louder, have been phased out and replaced with NeuroTechnology™. The significant cognitive benefits to NeuroTechnology™ include: *binaural processing* (two ears working together), *sound orientation* (ability to detect the source of incoming sounds with increased accuracy), *enhanced clarity of voices* (even soft speakers), automatic *adaptation to environment* (no more pushing buttons and adjusting volume), and *noise-cancellation* filtering of background noise to enhance hearing conversation in noisy environments (hearing better in crowded rooms, restaurants, etc.).

What is the primary benefit of NeuroTechnology™?

This answer is outlined in greater detail throughout the book. In summary, recent reports find that NeuroTechnology™ and the treatment of hearing loss can significantly improve quality of life, reduce the risk of developing dementia, and offer an increase in cognitive function. Yes, all of this can be achieved by treating your hearing loss.

How do I get started with NeuroTechnology™?

It's simple: Request an appointment with the local audiology clinic that sent you this book, or visit *www.ExcellenceinAudiology.org* to find a member-clinic in your area. Most clinics will offer a free initial consultation to see if you are a good candidate for hearing loss treatment.

Is getting traditional hearing aids still effective treatment for hearing loss?

For the majority of patients, traditional hearing aids will not effectively treat hearing loss or the symptoms of hearing loss, including tinnitus. Traditional hearing aids are volume-enhancing devices that may help certain people in very limited environments (e.g. conversing one-on-one in a room with *no* background noise). For patients needing to follow conversation in dynamic environments (e.g. sitting at a dinner table with family and friends, going out to a restaurant, sitting in a lecture hall or a place of worship, playing cards with others, etc.), NeuroTechnology™ will restore clarity and enhance speech even in background noise.

Can I use my insurance benefit and Flex-Spending with TreatmentFi™?

Yes. TreatmentFi™ is customized to meet your hearing, cognitive, and financial needs. With this program, any insurance benefit you may have can be deducted from your monthly payment. In addition, payment for the treatment of hearing loss can be paid for through the use of a Flexible Spending Account set up at your employer.

What if I need an emergency appointment before or after office hours?

(This answer is a bit longer than most because of the seriousness of some audiology emergencies)

Audiology emergencies most often fall in to one of two categories:

Sudden change in hearing

While rare, a sudden change in hearing can occur. This medical condition, known as *sudden-onset sensorineural hearing loss*, may occur in one, or both (even more rare), ears and is often associated with a virus (and sometimes occurs in tandem with an upper respiratory infection)

There is varying data on successful treatment protocols for this disorder; regardless, the key to potentially recovering hearing function requires seeking medical attention within 24–48 hours of initial symptoms.

Emergency related to the NeuroTechnology™

Broken or "non-functioning devices" may occur from time to time during your treatment. If there is any disturbance, such as lost domes, tight speaker wires, or irritation, call your hearing care provider's office as soon as possible to have them evaluate the urgency of the problem and schedule you to be seen accordingly. In the interim, here are helpful hints to remedy some of the problems that you may encounter until you can be seen in the office:

■ If a device is itching your ear, use some ear lotion included in your treatment package.

■ A device causing feedback or "squealing" can generally be worn until you are seen by our team. Call the office as soon as you notice this feedback or squealing so that we can schedule you to make a prescription change.

- A dome, earmold, or removable device that is not fitting well, is not to be worn until it can be properly adjusted at the office. Call the office as soon as possible to have your specialists make the adjustment for comfort and fit.

If you are experiencing an audiology emergency that can't wait for regular office hours, most audiology offices have a special number to call either before or after business hours. If you can wait until the office is open, most offices will have special emergency appointments set aside each day to help in these situations.

Can NeuroTechnology™ get wet?

Unlike traditional hearing aids that had no moisture resistance, most of today's NeuroTechnology™ comes with an IP57 rating for dust and moisture resistance. In lay terms, the "IP" stands for International Protection Rating and the "5" indicates the unit is Dust Protected (highest score is a 6 on this scale) and the "7" indicates the unit can be immersed in up to one meter of water (that is over three feet!). With that said—we continue to direct patients to not swim or bathe with their NeuroTechnology™.

Should I sleep with my NeuroTechnology™?

It is recommended to not sleep with your NeuroTechnology™ for three reasons:

1. Give your ear a rest—sleeping with the unit can cause discomfort to the pinna and side of the head.

2. It is easier for the unit to fall out when tossing and turning in bed and may get lost.

3. It will wear out the batteries in half the time of their intended lifespan if used 24 hours per day.

However, I do have patients that sleep with their NeuroTechnology™ for safety and personal reasons.

How do I regularly clean my NeuroTechnology™?

Like with cleaning your home…clean it a little each day and it won't become such a mess! Your specialist will help you understand daily and monthly routines for maintaining your NeuroTechnology™ at home. Use a lint free cloth and brush (typically provided at your first treatment appointment) to wipe down the unit every day. This will help prevent oils from the skin, dandruff, earwax, and other environmental dust from clogging the microphones and speaker over time. I also encourage my patients to change the "parts" once a month. This includes wax filters (designed to prevent earwax from entering the unit), domes (designed to securely hold the unit in the ear) and microphone filters (included on some NeuroTechnology™ options).

INTERVIEW WITH
DR. DANA DAY

Interviewed by John Melley

JOHN MELLEY: Hello and welcome to the program. Do you or a loved one have impaired hearing? Did you know hearing problems can lead social isolation and increase your risk for other health problems? Do you want to remain independent and live an active life as you age? Well, all of these can be affected by the quality of your hearing. If you or someone you care for has impaired hearing or you think you might, this is a program you want to pay attention to.

My guest today is Dr. Dana L. Day. And she's here to talk about hearing loss and what you can do about it to maintain a high quality of life. But before we begin my conversation with Dr. Day, let me tell you a little about her. Dr. Day began her training in Germany at Second General Regional Hospital serving not only our brave men and women and their families but also our NATO troops from all around Europe. And it was during this time in Germany that she discovered her love for and passion for the "dizzy" patient as well as those suffering from hearing disorders. She went on to hone her skills with the pediatric population at Boy's Town National Hospital before returning to Phoenix to start her audiology career.

Dr. Day was instrumental in the development of several balance and concussion centers throughout Phoenix including work with Barrow Neurological Institute. And Dr. Day is sought after for her expertise in hearing and balance, as well her work with the pediatric patient. She has written several articles, the most recent for the American Tinnitus Association and she is the owner of the multidisciplinary hearing and balance healthcare practice in Phoenix, Arizona Balance and Hearing Aids.

She has been a guest faculty at ASU and A.T. Still. She has been an instructor for concussion health webinars and courses. She's a member of the American Speech Language Hearing Association and the Academy of Doctors of Audiology. And she has provided hearing screenings, supervision and oversight for annual hearing screenings for Madison Simis Elementary School and provides education on noise and offers musician plugs to young musicians at the Arizona School for the Performing Arts.

And this is cool. She has provided musician ear protection at cost to ABHA to orchestra members. And on top of all of these, she is a member of the Grace Lutheran Church Council. She has time to sponsor the Sunnyslope High School Dance Team and manage a boy's soccer team. My goodness, Doctor! [Laughter] That is an awful lot. How are you? Thanks for coming to the program.

DR. DANA DAY: Well, thanks for having me. And after that wonderful introduction, I think I need to take a nap. But I'm here.

JOHN MELLEY: [Laughter] Well, you built the resume.

DR. DANA DAY: And I'm ready to go.

[Laughter]

JOHN MELLEY: That's great. You know, one thing I think our listeners would be interested in, you have such a broad background, an interesting background as well with your work over in Europe with the NATO troops and our men and women serving in Germany. But tell us, how did this whole story unfold for you? How did this become a passion of yours?

DR. DANA DAY: That's a very good question. I kind of—not kind of, I did come in through the back door, if you will. I grew up in a very small farming community in eastern Washington State, left there to come to Arizona State University because I am just not a cold weather person and decided I like the sunshine.

And it was there that I started my educational career, if you will, with education primarily in deaf education. And I was two years into the program in Public Law on 94-142 passed which is the law that mainstreams children into the regular classroom. And there was this fear that there would be no need for deaf educators. And at that time, I was taking my sign language classes in the speech and hearing department at ASU and I thought "Well, let me try this." And so, I went into that program, tried both speech and hearing, found my passion to be more in the hearing realm or audiology, if you will, and finished there.

Then went on for my masters at Colorado State University where I was a teaching assistant. And from there went on to get my doctorate back here in Arizona. Really kind of a roundabout way to get into the profession but it was when I really got to put my hands and my heart into the families and military personnel overseas is when I really grasp, this is really my passion. This is what I love to do.

JOHN MELLEY: What was it about hearing in particular that it really made you so passionate about it?

DR. DANA DAY: The beauty of sign language. And the ability to communicate with someone who otherwise couldn't hear verbally. That's kind of where I started with deaf education. And just the ability to communicate with these wonderful people.

And then it kind of moved more in a different realm as my career started taking off and I got to meet more and more people of all different ages, all different backgrounds and finding that no matter where they come from or what their background is or how old they are, hearing is such an instrumental, monumental part of being able to communicate. And the ability to communicate, to go in and buy a loaf of bread, to go into the bank, to go to your doctor's office, it's huge. More so then I believe anybody and that includes myself realizes until they actually get into this and start looking around them and saying, "You know, this isn't so easy for some people. But I can help them."

JOHN MELLEY: That's very, very cool. Believe or not, I am looking at the clock. We need to take a quick break. But when we come back, I'd like to talk a little bit more about how amazing our sense of hearing is. But also let's talk about how important it is to maintain what we have. So, let's talk about that when we come back, OK?

[Break]

JOHN MELLEY: Welcome back. My guest today is Dr. Dana L. Day and we are talking about the importance of hearing for communicating. I think hearing is a sense that we'd take for granted. Can you talk to us really about how important our hearing is, aside from just talking and hearing birds and listening to music and all that kind of stuff. Let's talk about hearing, our sense of hearing, how vital it is.

DR. DANA DAY: Well, I think you're right. Many of us take our hearing for granted, or we just say it's a part of aging, or if people just wouldn't mumble, or I don't like the way they build restaurants these days, or we can find all these different excuses, all of us can to make it as part of life, as part of aging that we are just going to lose our hearing and things are going to get more difficult. But it really isn't necessarily a part of aging. In fact, it has to do with the external factors that you bring in whether that be noise, medication effects, trauma, all these different things.

But once you lose the ability to understand or communicate or engage in an activity, they become socially isolated. They do not engage with their family, with their neighbors, with their church group, the things that were very, very important to them prior to all of these happening with their hearing. And usually, in most cases, it happens over time. And so, we might not notice it yesterday but today it was a little harder. Well, it's probably because I was in this situation listening or that situation listening. But it can also become very much a life altering condition in the sense of, again, if you socially isolate, you stop doing the things that you want to do. But when you go to your doctor, and you'd think he said or she said, take this twice a day when they said it twice a week.

So these are very important things that we don't think about on a regular basis. But it's very, very important. If you have family that lives away from you, so maybe not in the same town, they can't come visit all the time but you won't engage with your grandchildren or your children or your niece or nephew and you're unable to do that because it's difficult to understand them over the phone. The clarity isn't there. And so, it just becomes too hard to have those conversations. It's much of a reminder of what you can't do. And that is really a part of this conversation that I would like to let the listeners know. It doesn't need to happen. There are solutions for all different conditions of hearing loss that will allow you to re-engage in those activities that are the most important to you.

JOHN MELLEY: And that's very interesting. So, what you're saying is because it becomes difficult for some people to hear their loved ones and friends and family. They basically just kind of slowly shut down and just sit, withdraw from folks because they just can't understand them.

DR. DANA DAY: Correct. Correct.

JOHN MELLEY: That's sad.

DR. DANA DAY: It is sad. An activity that may have been very much a part of their lives, example, dinner with the family now becomes something that they put themselves in the corner because they can't understand what's going on. And they don't want to misinterpret things. And then it may become they don't even sit in the corner anymore, maybe they don't even go.

JOHN MELLEY: Or, you misunderstand something and you respond in a way that might not make sense and people start to look at you go, "I wasn't trying to be mean." They misunderstand you and it causes an argument or un-intended consequences, huh?

DR. DANA DAY: Correct. Correct.

JOHN MELLEY: Well, that's a lot to think about here. You would send some information over to our producer before the show and one of the things that jumped out at me was that hearing loss can lead to other health issues. And I wondered if we could talk about that.

DR. DANA DAY: Sure. One of the things that is not as common knowl-edge in the community, even in the medical commu-nity is what we call comorbidities that are associated with hearing loss. So, comorbidity is you may have this going on but it also can cause this.

You may have diabetes for example, and if you have diabetes you have a 40% greater risk of having a hearing loss because of the diabetes. So, those two we would say are comorbid, they work together. The diabetes is the primary diagnosis but it's creating the hearing loss which is the secondary diagnosis.

JOHN MELLEY: Wow. And why is that?

DR. DANA DAY: Well, in the case of diabetes, diabetes is a situation, as most of you know, which the pancreas does not produce the insulin that it needs to produce to metabolically keep our bodies going. So what happens is when you get too much sugar in the blood, it thickens and it damages the tiny capillaries of the nerve endings. So within the ear, we have those tiny capillaries. So, if most of our listeners have heard of neuropathy which is usually at the feet or hands, that's the tingling or the sharp needle pains because of that depletion of blood flow into those areas, the extremities. Well, the same thing can happen in the ears or the inner ear if you will.

So, you can have neuropathy of the inner ear because next to the brain, the inner ear demands the most oxygen and you get that through the blood flow. So, if you have thickening of the blood that causes these capillaries to become damage then they're not flowing that blood into that space. And therefore, the outer hair cells which is what we hear with start to deplete and die off. Just like in your fingers or in your toes or in your feet when you have the neuropathy in there just like those nerve endings are not firing and working like they should and therefore you're feeling the tingling or the sensation of the pins or needles.

JOHN MELLEY: So, instead of tingling in the ears, you're having a diminished amount of hearing.

DR. DANA DAY: Correct.

JOHN MELLEY: Yeah, this is so fascinating. It just shows that everything is connected, isn't it?

DR. DANA DAY: It is. It is.

JOHN MELLEY: Yeah. You know, I'm looking at the clock, we need to take a quick break but when we come back, let's talk some more about some of the other issues that can arise from a hearing loss, OK?

Welcome back. My guest today is Dr. Dana L. Day and just before the break, we were discussing how diabetes can affect hearing and result in a hearing loss. And there are also some other health implications from hearing loss, aren't there Doctor?

DR. DANA DAY: Yes, there is. And thank you for asking. Research studies and I think the one our listeners would be most concerned about is the link that Dr. Lin, out of Johns Hopkins University, has shown between hearing loss and cognitive decline or dementia.

In his research, he has found that there is a 40% to 60% greater risk to an individual in acquiring dementia with untreated hearing loss. So again, we're talking about that comorbidity.

And the reason for that is many people think we hear in our ears. But we really don't. We hear in our brain.

Sound waves come in, they bounce off the middle ear or the tympanic membrane or the ear drum and they vibrate the three bones, many people heard them in school as the anvil, hammer and stirrup.

JOHN MELLEY: Yup, I remember that.

DR. DANA DAY: Yes. And that vibrates that sound through the cochlea which is a snail-shaped structure and that sends those sound waves up the auditory nerve which is one of your 12 cranial nerves to the brain. And the brain makes sense of all these sound waves coming in. Now, at the level of the cochlea, we also hear different— we get different pitches and sounds so that's why the brain can figure out a P from an M, so mat versus pat, for example.

And we're stimulating the brain all the time with sounds around us so that we can make sense of our auditory environment. So, sitting here right now I'm in a quiet room but there's a window next to me and there is a fire station so every now and then I hear a fire truck go by. I can process the fire truck is going by but it doesn't interrupt my conversation with you or with your listeners because our brain is being inundated all the time with sounds and we have to decide what we're going to listen to and what we're not going to listen to.

JOHN MELLEY: Kind of tune it out.

DR. DANA DAY: Exactly. But we still need to know what's going on around us. And so, we're stimulating that area of the brain constantly from the corpus callosum to the hippocampus all the way up to the temporal and cortical levels. So we're always stimulating that. But if we have a hearing loss, that stimulation decreases.

We don't get the same energy or auditory energy into the brain that we used to. And so, the brain just kind of decides to disregard or die off, if you will. And that's a bad term because it doesn't actually die but it can start to shrink and atrophy over time. And so, there are a lot of things that go into that but hearing is one of them and it is a primary one of them. Many times we're taking earlier about people saying, it's just part of aging. People just need to talk louder. I just need to turn the TV up louder. That's really not going to help the situation because it doesn't help get those subtle sounds and the clarity of those subtle sounds to the brains. The brain can still remain active and figure out what is all going on around me? Was that somebody that just walked by my front door? Did the phone ring in the other room? How can I find my car when I beep it and I can't hear it, those types of things, in a parking lot?

JOHN MELLEY: Yeah.

DR. DANA DAY: So, those are the types of things that we really don't think about on a daily basis but that are very, very important to keep our brains active and alive and working the way they did 20 years ago or 30 years ago.

JOHN MELLEY: Sure. And then that's fascinating. I'm also thinking that it might be personal safety issue. I mean if you're crossing the crosswalk or something like that and you don't hear a car coming up behind you or a person coming up behind you or something like that.

DR. DANA DAY: Yeah.

JOHN MELLEY: I can imagine that that would—it just puts us at greater risk all around.

DR. DANA DAY: It does.

JOHN MELLEY: Yeah. It really is kind of a situation of use it or lose it as everything else. You've got to stimulate the brain or else it just sort of says, "Yeah, OK, we don't need to do this anymore."

DR. DANA DAY: Right. Exactly. Exactly. We want to maintain a good cognitive health throughout our lives and we do that through puzzles and Sudoku and crosswords puzzles and all these games that are out there now online.

JOHN MELLEY: Right.

DR. DANA DAY: But we also need to maintain it through what we're bringing in auditorily because that is so important to the brain to stimulate those areas. There are so many shared pathways in the brain that the auditory system needs to be able to get to all those pathways and innervate them so that that cognitive health remains strong, active and productive.

JOHN MELLEY: Now, I have a question for you. Is there a way to—can they quantify like what percentage of the brain is actually used for hearing? I mean I know the visual cortex is in the back of your skull but I mean can we say like if you, your hearing uses X percent of your brain's area or something like that.

DR. DANA DAY: I think if you want it to really quantitative, you'd have to look at each one. So, I'm going to take one of the areas we call the corpus callosum. And the corpus callosum takes auditory information from one side of the brain and moves it over to the other side.

So you have what we call dichotic listening. So if you're at a cocktail party and someone is on your right, and someone is behind you, and someone is on your left, and someone is in front of you, you're able to take in the information but you can bring in what you're wanting to listen to for instance.

And the area of the corpus callosum of the brain is responsible for over 90% of auditory transfer. That's what it—it does visual transfer, somatosensory which is feel or touch transfer. But its primary goal is for auditory transfer so you can hear all those things, block out what you don't want to listen to, listen to what you do, integrate information so that you know that little Johnny just fell over here and I need to go attend to him type of thing.

JOHN MELLEY: Got you.

DR. DANA DAY: And that's just one part of the brain. So, then there's other parts that are responsible that taking auditory information are responsible for learning and daily function, the fight or flight response. When you hear something you have to know, do I need to get away from this situation, do I need to engage in this situation type of thing? So the brain is just such a wonderful thing that we have been given.

JOHN MELLEY: Yeah.

DR. DANA DAY: And it takes in so much and so much is integrated together and weaved through it. We need to—if your eyes go bad, for instance, we go get glasses. We don't think anything about that. If our prescription changes, we change our prescription. But when our hearing starts to go, we say, "Well, we'll just turn it up." Or, "We just won't go there because I can't hear very well." We don't really address it the same way but we need to because auditorily, it's just as important if not more so for brain health that you hear all those things.

JOHN MELLEY: My producer is waving madly at me. I'm so engrossed in this conversation, we have to take another break but when we comeback, let's talk some more about this. It almost like our—the corpus callosum, it sounds like our almost our own internal surround sound system. [Laughter]

DR. DANA DAY: It is. That's a very good way of looking at it.

JOHN MELLEY: OK. But let's talk some more about how important this is and maybe why some folks are a little embarrassed. And I want to tell you something when we come back too.

Welcome back. My guest today is Dr. Dana L. Day and we are talking about our sense of hearing. And Doctor, this has been fascinating because like you said earlier, in the program most folks think, "Ah, so I can't hear as well, I just turn it up." Or, "I'll sit in the different part of the restaurant so I can hear better." Or, "Yeah, I just won't go to the party because it's too loud." And there's a lot more to it than that.

Your hearing can be affected by a diabetes and you were discussing was that hearing loss can lead to dementia. And you've made the analogy of if we had a vision loss, we'd go and get glasses. But for some reason, there seems to be a bit of a hang up when it comes to out hearing and putting that off. Do you think that's because there's some sort of stigma or that subconsciously, perhaps we know how important our hearing is to us and we might be in some sort of denial about it.

DR. DANA DAY: I think it's probably a bit of both. But if we go back to the stigma that I think that's probably stronger side of that. And I say that because well we have and I have patients that are under the age of 10 but have a hearing loss. That isn't a big high percentage. But if we looked at that same percentage of children in the schools that have to wear glasses, I think we would see a higher percent of those wearing glasses. So it's kind of in a way more socially acceptable, if you will.

JOHN MELLEY: Glasses are?

DR. DANA DAY: Yeah. And they've even become a fashion statement. I remember my roommate years ago used to wear glasses as part of her outfit, as an accessory even though she didn't need glasses. So, you've got the glasses without needed correction.

JOHN MELLEY: Prescription? Yeah, yeah.

DR. DANA DAY: So, it's kind of like we've made it socially acceptable and to some degree, "Oh! That's really neat. I really like your glasses." But you don't have a lot of people saying "I really like our hearing aids. It's really neat. Oh, is that—look at that color I just love it." We don't have that in our society.

JOHN MELLEY: No. Yeah, yeah, yeah.

DR. DANA DAY: So we, as a society, I believe see hearing aid as I'm getting old. I'm aging. But we don't see it the same way with glasses. So, that I believe is probably why people aren't as eager to go out and get hearing aids as they would for the glasses. And then other thing too is just like when you have the vision problem, many times your vision goes right away, in the sense of I used to be able to see that and now I can't. So, it must be, "Oh if I go this way or if I go this way or if I put on the readers that I can get at the drug store, oh, now I can see." Your hearing though usually goes subtly too, little bit, little bit, and little bit. And so what we find ourselves doing is as I mentioned before, "So they radio just gets a little bit louder or the volume on the TV gets a little bit louder." Or you tell your spouse, "Listen, if I'm in the other room, don't talk to me, I can't hear you." Right?

JOHN MELLEY: [Laughter] Oh yeah.

DR. DANA DAY: You need to come in here and stand in front of me so I can hear you because there's all this stuff going on when in fact, or the great comment and we've all said this, "I can't hear through walls." Right?

JOHN MELLEY: Right.

DR. DANA DAY: And so, it's a little bit different I think as we perceive it. But I think the biggest perception is glasses are OK, hearing aids are "I'm getting old".

JOHN MELLEY: Yeah.

DR. DANA DAY: Kind of like the cane, you know?

JOHN MELLEY: Yeah. Well, I have a confession to make. And one of the reasons why I asked the question and the reason why I laughed so loudly when you said "Don't go in the other room and talk" is that I've recently having spent more than 20 years in a recording studio with headphones and been a musician for a good portion of my life and playing in ensembles and playing the drums and all that kind of stuff. I am getting treated for hearing loss. And it's interesting—and I will admit I felt like, "Oh gosh, here we go. I'm only 51." But I'm thinking you know my dad he's 82 and he has hearing aids. And so, that's what older folks do.

DR. DANA DAY: Right.

JOHN MELLEY: So, I understand that feeling but what do you say to that person? What would you say to me, if you said,

"John, you know what? You've really got—you've got a hearing loss and it really should be treated because of all the things that you had said before there's an increase risk for dementia." And I said, "You know, well Dr. Day, I'm only 51." What do you say?

DR. DANA DAY: Age is a number. [Laughter] No. I would say to any patient that comes in that is in need of amplification or hearing aid to help in their understanding of. It's not about age. It's not about what it will look like. It's about engagement. We want you to remain active and engaged in your community, whatever that community looks like. And we want all of our patients, you included, you're not my patient but all of those with hearing loss, to experience all the wonderful things that come at them auditorily because there are some wonderful things that the orchestra, the favorite music playing, hearing the difference between the keys on the piano, wonderful things that we get to listen to our grandchildren, our children. So, we want that to stay the same. We want that enjoyment in our live and in all of our lives and on our patient's live regardless of what age you are.

And because you are 51 and you are very active, this is not the time to pull back or disengage from those activities. This is the time to enjoy them. So, the hearing aid will just—or aids, will just allow you to do that. They will allow you the clarity and this is very important, technology increases and I know we're going to talk about this later but as technology increases it's not about just making things louder, it's making things clearer. And it's the clarity that we need. And we want to make sure that when you go in to a meeting or you go in to your recording studio, that everything is clear for you. That your job is just as easy as it was before the hearing loss that there's no anxiety. There's no wondering if you heard it right. There's just the pleasure of doing your profession.

JOHN MELLEY: Right. You know, it's interesting that you talk about the technology. I want to talk about that but we have to take another quick break. Let's talk about that and how the technology has improved over the years.

Welcome back. My guest today is Dr. Dana L. Day and just before the break, we were talking about—I made a true confession Doctor, I told you that I am currently getting treated for hearing loss but that's due to almost a quarter of a century of recording studios and loud music and rock concerts without hearing protection. [Laughter] If I only had known then what I only had known now, right?

DR. DANA DAY: Yes. In hindsight, we're all brilliant aren't we?

JOHN MELLEY: Yeah. But we talked about how diabetes can affect your hearing and how a hearing loss can increase your risk of dementia by you said, the research indicates by 40% to 60% increase of risk?

Basically, it's a situation of your brain is not getting stimulated enough because you're not hearing the different frequencies of sound that we are able to hear when we, I guess when we're born with our hearing.

But you had mentioned before the break that there are some other health concerns that hearing losses can create. What would those be?

DR. DANA DAY: One of them is aging, simple aging. And what we find is hearing loss due to aging affects men more than women. And one of the reasons is men tend to be in more high risk auditory positions than women. And you're an example. You are a percussionist, a drummer, you went to a lot of concerts, you didn't wear ear protection. Many men work in industrial sites or drive large heavy equipment and may not use ear protection. So, aging can be one of those factors.

And part of the dementia and that number that 40, 60 is would include cognitive decline. You can have cognitive decline and not dementia or not Alzheimer's I mean there's degrees of it. So, you have cognitive decline which is associated with the change in the brain structure because of the reduced volume or auditory information to the brain.

And another one that we don't think about is the risk of falls. A hearing loss diminishes the spatial awareness or reduces attention capacity which would increase the fall risk. So, when I talk about spatial awareness, it's things like where your body is in space, in that room, if you will.

You might be walking down the hall and you hear something and you go to turn and you turned too soon or you turned too late and so you hit against the wall.

Also, the inner ear where the cochlea is located also contains the balance mechanism, if you will. I always call it the gyroscope of our body and they're connected. So, if you have reduced hearing due to damage in the cochlea, you can also have some reduced—not always but you can also have reduced responses in that inner ear space or those balance canals. And so, you're high risk for falls. And that is also very much an increase and we know that that is becoming a health crisis in the United States.

Number one, if you are over the age of 75 and you fall in your home, there is a very good chance eight out of 10 that you will not be able to return to your home due to a broken hip or injuries that you sustained. And we also know that billions of our medical health care dollars are being spent every year on patients that fall, whether they fall at home or in their—outside of the home, at the assisted living community, wherever it is and so this has become a health crisis within the United States. And it has been brought to the attention as we need to do something about this. And so, we're all looking at ways to reduce risk of falls and one of those ways is to make sure that you have proper hearing. And that's usually through the use of hearing aids. So, that's another one a lot of people don't think about.

JOHN MELLEY: No. Yeah, I wouldn't have thought about it but I do know that our balance center is in our ears, that part of the head anyway. Huh! You mentioned something about changes in the size of the brain structurally due to cognitive decline. Is this something that if you get proper treatment that you can reverse?

DR. DANA DAY: Yes. And it's not just if you get proper treatment with hearing aids, it's again what—if you have that hearing aids and you're getting that auditory information. And vision loss, if you're making sure that your glasses are correct and you're getting that visual stimulus. And if you have difficulty with what we call somatosensory or tactile information making sure that you understand that when things are hot, pull away versus keeping your hand there because you can't feel it. So, all of those things our brain takes in and makes sense of our world around us. And hearing is very important part of that as well.

JOHN MELLEY: Are there any other health issues?

DR. DANA DAY: Yes, two others that maybe are audience haven't thought about and that is kidney disease. So the kidneys are filter if you will. And they filter out toxins of our body but 54% of American adults with chronic kidney disease, they have higher probability of hearing loss because those toxins aren't filtered out of the kidneys as we would like or hope.

So, as part of their annual routine, just as with the diabetic, an annual hearing test is really recommended so that those can be monitored and if in fact intervention is needed, it's done quickly and expeditiously to maintain good brain health.

And then finally, heart disease, we have found again, medical community through research has found that if you get a hearing test in this show what we call a low frequency loss, that has been found to be tied to heart disease and so that could be the precursor to you seeing a cardiologist if that's the case. But if you already have heart disease, again, due to inner ear sensitivity, the blood flow we talked about earlier and that being disrupted with the heart disease they tend to have—those that have heart disease tend to have a higher comorbidity rate for hearing loss as well.

So, our hearing is tied to all of these things, diabetes, aging, dementia, cognitive decline, kidney disease, risk of falls, vision loss and heart disease. So, we really should not be ignoring it. We really should say, "You know what? This is really important to me and it's important to my health and it's important to my livelihood and my ability to age the way I want, so I'm going to take of this. I'm going to go see my audiologist and I'm going to take care of this." And that I think is the strongest message I would like to send out to people today is it's OK. You're not alone. It's not OK to do nothing, do something.

JOHN MELLEY: Right. It's a lot more than just saying, huh?

DR. DANA DAY: Uh-huh.

JOHN MELLEY: It has a lot of far reaching consequences than just saying that a lot and annoying people.

DR. DANA DAY: Mm-hmm.

JOHN MELLEY: It really has a life or death implications, don't it?

DR. DANA DAY: Yes, it does.

JOHN MELLEY: Yeah. We need to take another quick break but when we come back, let's talk about how technology has improved over the years and how they might lessen the sting in terms of "Oh my gosh, I've got hearing aids!" [Laughter] Is that OK?

DR. DANA DAY: That's great. I'd love to.

PART 2 OF THE INTERVIEW

JOHN MELLEY: Welcome back. My guest today is Dr. Dana L. Day and we are talking about treating hearing loss and how important that is. And in the last portion of our conversation, you talked about heart disease, high risk for falls, kidney disease, diabetes, dementia, cognitive decline, a whole host of health issues. Are there any others?

DR. DANA DAY: One of the things that our listeners maybe have heard about or very much aware of is called tinnitus or tinnitus, you can pronounce it either way. And that's any type of what I call head noise, a buzzing, a ringing, a hissing noise in their ears or their head. Sometimes they can isolate it to it's in my ears and sometimes they say it's in the middle of my head. And many people have tinnitus, simply because of the hearing loss that they have. Common theory of tinnitus is that you have hair cells in the inner ear that work to take that sound wave that comes in and then change it to different pitches and sounds or frequencies. So that you have high pitch sounds like the PHs and Fs that you can hear versus the low pitch which are your vowels, A, E, I, O, U.

The idea is that when the hair cells become damaged because of noise exposure, ototoxicity which is medications that are toxic to the oto- ear system or trauma, head trauma or other things as well. Those hair cells pull away or become damaged but they still fire and that's where you're hearing the tinnitus or the ringing. Now, this is one theory. We're not totally sure what causes tinnitus but this is one of the accepted theories that it might be. Many times in those cases as long as you're just not in quiet, you do fine.

It's when you go to lay down at night, it's really quiet and then you hear it and then it becomes a problem. And when people go to their doctors and say, "I have ringing in my ears." They're basically told, "Well, you'll just have to live with it or don't ever be in quiet." So that's not a really good solution for everyone.

JOHN MELLEY: No.

DR. DANA DAY: And they work for some but it doesn't work for everyone. So, in our clinic, we have taken the approach of what is out there and available that is legitimate, meaning the science is behind it that would help our patients with the ringing in their ears or the tinnitus. Now, some of them by simply putting a hearing aid on and increasing those higher frequencies and the higher pitch sounds, increasing those tones that they can't hear, it masks meaning that it brings in sounds so that you don't hear the internal sounds—things—sounds from the external environment so they don't hear the internal environment.

So the problem is at night when you take them off. It might still be there. But that from 90% of the patients will work just fine. For some, we have to add what we call a masker, meaning it's a sound kind of like the wind blowing, if you will, that goes in there and it just kind of quiets the sound internally for them so that they can calm down. They're not so anxious and go on throughout their day. Many of those patients when they take their hearing aids off at night or their maskers and then will use an external device like waves or the ocean or the fan running at night.

JOHN MELLEY: Like some white noise or something like that. Yeah.

DR. DANA DAY: Yes, exactly, white noise. But there are a few percentage, about 2% to 4% of those patients with tinnitus that it's debilitating. No matter what they do, it's there.

They can't sleep. They can't eat. They just can't function because of the ringing in their ears. And those patients require a little bit more aggressive technology and treatment. So, instead of playing a hearing aid with a masker on, we may do things such as tinnitus retraining therapy, cognitive feedback therapy and now, there are devices out there that they can wear at night to help calm that stimulus to the brain and we are one of the sites here in Phoenix, Arizona which provides this to that patient population.

And so, I think that when you're talking about tinnitus, one needs to remember that it's not a one-shot deal. If this doesn't work, you just live with it. If this doesn't work, you just live with it. Or, you need a hearing aid and then that will take care of it. Sometimes you need both, sometimes you need some type of therapy and the hearing aid. I would invite everyone that's listening to really think about this and if they have tinnitus and it's debilitating, it's causing problems in their sleep patterns to consult with an audiologist who have more than one solution for their tinnitus. And I also would like to encourage any of our listeners who are veterans. This is the number one reason veterans go to a VA hospital is ringing in their ears.

JOHN MELLEY: Wow.

DR. DANA DAY: And it can be for some who have been involved in bomb blast that had acoustic trauma can be one of those situations where it's—it can be borderline debilitating for them. So, if you are a veteran and you're listening to this, visit your VA. Ask them what other solutions there are. If they don't have those, use your veteran's choice because there's a wonderful study with the Portland VA in collaboration with the Cedar-Sinai Hospital that have looked at different therapy methods to help them in the realm of their tinnitus that goes beyond just fitting them with the hearing aid.

JOHN MELLEY: Now, that's great information to have and I'm sure source of hope for some of our vets that are dealing with that.

DR. DANA DAY: Yes, I hope so.

JOHN MELLEY: Yeah. Welcome back. My guest today is Dr. Dana L. Day and we have been talking about the importance of hearing and treating hearing loss and how hearing loss has far reaching implications to our overall health and our social interaction with those that we care about. Earlier in our conversation, you talked about how the stigma of people have with hearing aids versus people who might go get glasses that you know glasses people sometimes just wear them for a fashion statement and that glasses tend to be more accepted in society because they seem to be everywhere. You know you can go and buy them at I don't know at drug store or wholesale club or whatever, in addition to your optometrist.

But hearing aids aren't as necessarily as readily available although we are starting to see some things, you see those ads on TV where somebody is holding something and then you know there's this guy and there are two women over on the other side of the football fields saying, "Oh isn't he so cute?" And he's just shaking his head like "Yeah, they're talking about me." We're not talking about that kind of stuff are we? [Laughter]

DR. DANA DAY: No, of course not. [Laughter]

JOHN MELLEY: We're talking about sounds a little more sophisticated than that, I would think. But you know, I mean it's a question because that's what people are seeing. So, talk to me about how technology has progressed over the years for hearing devices.

DR. DANA DAY: Well, that is a really great question. Technology in every realm has progressed over the years. So, before we get into that conversation, I wanted to make sure to clarify something that you said. You're right, hearing aids are popping up more and more at our drug stores online at wholesale stores, member clubs.

JOHN MELLEY: Yeah.

DR. DANA DAY: But I think it's very important to understand and make the distinction between what's popping up in areas and what that actually means. When I first started, hearing aid was basically an amplifier.

JOHN MELLEY: OK.

DR. DANA DAY: We've all seen the comics or the diagrams of the ear horn that somebody would put up to their ear. And we've seen the one where people would wear them on their chest, the big boxes. Well, those were amplifiers. And even when I started in this profession, with a few exceptions of just being able to change what we called the frequency pattern, they were amplifiers and that's what they did. They amplified all the sound.

And so, I think the biggest shift in technology that we're seeing is we've gone from analogue, meaning if

I turned it up one, it turns the volume one across the board. If I turned it up two, it turns the volume up two. And when you go into your local store and you see this instrument, you need to ask yourself is this an amplifier? Or is this a hearing aid that's going to help me? And there is big distinction between the two.

Hearing aids now like I said have moved from analogue to digital. And the digital hearing aid allows us as audiologist to computer program, a chip within the hearing aid so that we can say, OK, when you get into noise, we don't want that background noise to be as prominent as the person in front of you. So, we are going to make sure that the microphone direction is going to—I used to say wherever you're looking. And then that was our first shift, the directional mic.

And then we go to all these different other shifts. And now, we're up to a point it's such a wonderful time to be in this profession right now because the hearing instruments or hearing aids that we're now being able to work with provide so many options to the wearers that they didn't have before. Options meaning it improve clarity because we can connect it to your phone whether it be an iPhone or Android. So you can use your phone as an amplifier, if you will. So, you can stick your phone in the middle of the table at a restaurant and the phone picks up only the people at your table and it goes directly, that sound goes directly to your hearing aids. And so that noise behind you, of the table that's having the birthday party and singing and laughing.

You can still have a wonderful dinner and conversation with your guest or your family at your table. Win noise, you can still ride your bike and not worry about this terrible noise going through your hearing aids and wanting to take them off but can't because you need to hear the car coming behind you.

It's just been a huge leap in technology and I can't think of a better time to be in audiology in this field because we have so many more options available to us but the hearing aids are only as good as the person that's fitting them. And so, if you get something that's over the counter and it's an amplifier and it does what you want it to do. That's great. But keep in mind that is not a hearing aid. That is an amplifier.

So, if you really need the technology that increases the sound and the clarity that's going to go to the brain and keep the brain health strong, you really need to see the audiologist that can show you all of the new technology out there. And so you the wearer, what is available to you and let the wearer make that decision. And since we're on that subject, you mentioned that you just recently got new hearing aids. I'm curious what is something that you found surprising when you actually got fit with the hearing aids?

JOHN MELLEY: Well, I'll tell you, it has been an interesting adjustment and I have very, very—despite the fact that I have a hearing loss, I also have picky hearing, because that's what I do, I work with sound. So I have been an interesting patient. But I will say that the first thing that happened when I went home with them was that my wife noticed that I wasn't talking as loudly at the dinner table.

DR. DANA DAY: Mm-hmm. Yes.

JOHN MELLEY: You know, I wasn't speaking so loudly that I was trying to hear myself which as a voice person has direct implications on liability to be able to perform for an extended period of time. I have less wear and tear and fatigue on my voice because I'm not talking as loudly.

DR. DANA DAY: Right.

JOHN MELLEY: And it's interesting—the reaction that I have I work in a radio station and people have started to notice them. And for a while, people didn't even know that I had them. They're that small. They're not those big things that you know you kind of think of. The interesting thing is people like, "Wow, you've already got a hearing loss? Well, I'm glad I don't really have that." And they're yelling at me. And I'm thinking, I want to turn the volume down but I can't because they don't have a volume control, it's coming out of very loud.

DR. DANA DAY: Right.

JOHN MELLEY: And I'm saying, "I think you do, you just don't know it yet because you're yelling." And I've noticed that— I've noticed the clarity with the higher end of things like sibilance and Ts and what we call fricatives which are Vs and Fs, those sounds, the fricatives because of the friction with the teeth on the lower lip. I'm getting too technical, but Bs versus Vs and Ms versus Ns and things of that nature. So, I've noticed that and my wife can actually be in the living room while I'm in the kitchen and she can say something and I'll for the most part get it you know. So, that's been good. And one of the things that she said to me was after I told her yeah, I mean I was—I was really kind of bummed out when I found out that I had the hearing loss, really, to be honest with you.

I was like, oh, man. And I wasn't always stupid with the hearing. I mean I wore hearing protection when I play the drums, if I cut the grass. I'm always wearing hearing protection using any machine or anything like that I have always used hearing protection you know, for as far back as I can remember. But when I was younger, I didn't and when I was in the band rooms I didn't. That's why I was interested in your work with the symphony in the youth orchestras etcetera because you know you're in a band room in a school, they're not necessarily acoustically treated, there's four walls and those sounds are vibrating in that small space. And I know some damage happen even going back into high school with some of that.

DR. DANA DAY: Right.

JOHN MELLEY: And I was in marching bands with the big drum lines and all that kind of stuff. And so—but I was bummed out you know, I'm not going to lie. I'm noticing different things. I've noticed—the first day I had them when I left the doctor's office, it happened to be raining and the sound of the rain on the car was different, as the drops hit the car. And then other thing is as I have been rewatching a television program that I really like and I've noticed that I'm picking up little subplots and storylines that I've watched the show a number of times and I never really put it into context or comprehension before. I was like, "Oh my gosh, I never noticed that before."

And I'm not watching subtitles anymore. And I'm saying so it's adding new dimensions to the storyline that I'm interested in and I think, "Oh my gosh, I was unaware of what I wasn't aware of!" if that makes sense.

DR. DANA DAY: Absolutely.

JOHN MELLEY: You don't know what you're missing. I think that's an interest—so...

DR. DANA DAY: You don't know what you don't know exactly.

JOHN MELLEY: You don't know what you don't know. So that's been my experience. As a matter of fact, I was talking with somebody the other day and I got into the shower with them.

DR. DANA DAY: Yes.

JOHN MELLEY: And I—that hadn't happened before. And you know I was like they say you know take them—don't wear them in the shower.

DR. DANA DAY: Mm-hmm.

JOHN MELLEY: That won't be good idea. But I thought, OK, I have become accustomed to this now because I didn't even know I had them on.

DR. DANA DAY: Exactly. And you wouldn't be the first person to come to me and I say, "I wore them into the shower." No.

JOHN MELLEY: I did. I rub my head and I was like, "Oh no!" I had to grab and put them on the towel and all that kind of stuff and I hope everything is fine with them. But that's the other interesting is they're pretty tough these little two head keys. So that has been my experience. You know we have to take another break but when we come back, let's—I did you know what before—you're going to have to wait. I'm going to take a break in a minute.

DR. DANA DAY: OK.

JOHN MELLEY: And I'm not talking to you, I'm talking to my producer. One question I wanted to ask you with regard—you mentioned amplifiers.

DR. DANA DAY: Mm-hmm.

JOHN MELLEY: If you just get an amplifier versus this technology that you're talking about, it occurs to me that part of the reason I have a hearing loss is because I was exposed to louder noises.

If it's just an amplifier, are you at an increased risk for further damaging your hearing just by getting an amplifier? And can you damage your hearing with the hearing aid? You know how like people say when you get glasses you're going to get a stronger prescription down the road because your eyes are just going to get weaker? Is that what happens with hearing aids? Can we talk about what when we come back?

DR. DANA DAY: Sure, absolutely.

JOHN MELLEY: All right. Welcome back. My guest today is Dr. Dana L. Day and we have been talking about hearing loss and protecting our hearing and how important our hearing is to us in general. Not just because we can't hear people and going, "Huh? What?" But it has far reaching implications for our overall health. And Doctor, we were talking about the technology and just before the break, you mentioned some hearing devices are just amplifiers versus some of this new high tech stuff that you can really only get when you go to a qualified audiologist such as yourself. And I was concerned about if you just get the amplifier, can you put yourself at risk for more hearing loss? And do some of the hearing devices that you work with by wearing them can you increasing your hearing loss by wearing them? What's the difference?

DR. DANA DAY: Very good question. For the hearing aids that we have in our office and all audiologists have, we have the ability to tap the amount of volume or sound that can come in through the hearing aid. In other words, if you have a mild hearing loss, we're never going to let anything get amplified above 80 decibels, for example.

If you have a severe to profound hearing loss, you'll need more amplification. So, we won't go anything above you know maybe 120 decibels because they need that much in because of those damaged hair cells. But no, a hearing aid programmed and set properly will not create additional hearing loss.

Other things could, if your health history changes, your medications, those types of things. With regards to the amplifiers, the ones that are currently being sold that you can just go pick up over the counter, they are by design through the FDA are supposed to be able to tap as well so that your limited to same amount that comes in. However, there are no regulations behind that.

So, to say that if you put an amplifier in and you accidentally turn it up too high and then a fire cracker goes off next to your ear, you'll probably get some damage.

JOHN MELLEY: Wow. Yeah.

DR. DANA DAY: Because there's no suppression of that sound. So you've got the loud sound coming in to a loud amplifier.

JOHN MELLEY: That makes sense. You can't say that it won't but you can't say that it will either, I get it.

DR. DANA DAY: Correct.

JOHN MELLEY: OK. We talked about how going to a qualified audiologist such as yourself that you can program these new hearing devices specifically for each, not just each person but for each year, right?

DR. DANA DAY: Correct. Uh-huh.

JOHN MELLEY: Huh. That's interesting. I didn't think about that. You know, one of the things that people talk about though and I've heard this is the cost of some of these hearing devices. So, how do you address that issue?

DR. DANA DAY: I am not going to lie to any of your listeners. Hearing aids can be expensive and are expensive. But again, it's not like your eyeglasses and your lenses where you can change every year. Your hearing aid, once it's programmed should last you for a good four or five, six even beyond years. And then also during that time, you get the service behind it, the warranty behind it. So, you need to kind of look at the investment that you're making as an investment on your hearing and your health that's going to cover you through five years.

So if you broke it down that way, and you look at the monthly cost, you're looking at far less than that initial "Whoa!" It's kind of like when you go to get a car. And you look at the car and you're like, "I don't have that kind of money. I can't buy this high end." But then when they come out and say, "But we can finance it for this. So you'd lease it for this."

"OK, that's make more sense on the budget." And for some places out there you can do that. And so, cost should really not be a factor, what should be a factor is how effective the hearing aids are going to be for you. Is the technology going to allow for neural plasticity, good neural health, again, brain health? And keep in mind that depending on where you go in our clinic, get free care in the sense of after the warranty is for the life of the hearing aid. So, tubing breaks or gets wet in the shower or those that you bring it in, we fix it. We have something for you to take home with you in case we have to send it in. So, I really think, when you're looking at this, you should look at it as a long-term investment in your health.

JOHN MELLEY: And I think you have to ask yourself, what's expensive? I mean heart disease, dementia, diabetes, high risk of falls those all have a heck of a lot bigger price tag attached to them than hearing devices. And as a person who has gone through this at this point, I can tell you that yeah, you go, huh, wow! But then you have to stop and think it's like, "Well, all right, how much do I spend on coffee every day?" Or, you're getting two basically high powered microcomputers for your head. [Laughter]

DR. DANA DAY: Right. Exactly.

JOHN MELLEY: You know. I mean so I heard somebody say something once and it made a lot of sense to me. If it's important to you, you will figure it out. You'll find a way to do it.

DR. DANA DAY: And we do that every day and things that we feel like you said is important to us.

JOHN MELLEY: Yeah. You know what Doctor? It looks like we have a phone call, let's go ahead and take that, OK?

DR. DANA DAY: OK.

JOHN MELLEY: Hi, who am I speaking with please?

ANNE: Hi there, this is Anne?

JOHN MELLEY: Hi Anne, how are you today?

ANNE: I am good.

JOHN MELLEY: Great. Are you a patient of Dr. Day's?

ANNE: I am indeed.

JOHN MELLEY: Tell us why you went to her practice and how did she help you out?

ANNE: Oh, she's helped out in numerous ways. Initially, I went to her for balance testing. I had symptoms that no doctor or other specialist could diagnose.

JOHN MELLEY: Huh, OK.

ANNE: Once I went to Dr. Day for the testing. She was able to diagnose me and get me situated so that my symptoms were more under control.

JOHN MELLEY: Oh, that's great.

ANNE: Yes. And it is and Dana has helped with my personal hearing issues and I've had over the years several different hearing aids dispensed by Dr. Day and/or her associates. And I can't say enough about the high quality of care and the knowledge level of everybody in the office. Dr. Day and her associates treated my elderly father who could have been a challenge to deal with but they made it quite easy and painless and he was thrilled with his experience as well.

JOHN MELLEY: Oh, that's terrific.

ANNE: Yeah.

JOHN MELLEY: Those dads can be a bit of challenge at times, can't they? [Laughter]

ANNE: Indeed he was very much of a challenge and I was thrilled with how they treated him with such dignity and with the outcome of him being able to hear us thereafter.

JOHN MELLEY: Well, that's wonderful. Would you recommend Dr. Day's practice to others?

ANNE: Without a doubt, yes.

JOHN MELLEY: Excellent. Is there anything else that you'd like to share with us?

ANNE: They are honest beyond honest and easy to get an appointment with, and above all, highly, highly professional.

JOHN MELLEY: That's wonderful. Well, Anne, I want to thank you for taking some time out of your day to share your thoughts with us.

ANNE: Sure. You're welcome.

JOHN MELLEY: Doctor, they sound thrilled.

DR. DANA DAY: Yes, they do and I'm so happy that they are thrilled. That really is why we do what we do at Arizona Balance and Hearing Aids.

JOHN MELLEY: That's great. It looks like we have another call. Hi, who am I speaking with please?

TOM: Tom Crow.

JOHN MELLEY: Hi, Tom. How are you today, sir?

TOM: I'm well, thank you.

JOHN MELLEY: Are you a patient of Dr. Day's?

TOM: I am.

JOHN MELLEY: Why did you go see her and what was your experience like?

TOM: Well, I went to see her on a recommendation and I was looking for hearing aids. And I knew I needed to see a competent audiologist. And so that's what led me to seeing her and in terms of my experience it has been excellent for a variety of reasons. They're pretty much always available. They take time to listen to you. You need your hearing aids reprogrammed from time to time they do that willingly and without charge. And so, my experience across the board has been outstanding.

JOHN MELLEY: Excellent. Now, did you know that you had had a hearing loss prior to visiting her practice? Or, is that something that you got diagnosed there?

TOM: Well, I knew I had a hearing loss but I didn't know the extent of it. You know, you pick up the fact that you're not hearing as well as you should. But the formal diagnosis and the hearing test was one that they conducted.

JOHN MELLEY: Excellent. Now, would you recommend her practice to others?

TOM: Without qualifications.

JOHN MELLEY: If there's one last thing that you want to leave with our listeners today what would that be?

TOM: Well, I guess it would be trust. You need to believe that the person you're dealing with is competent, that they're dealing with you honestly and straightforwardly. And that they are doing their best to address your problem and so that's what they bring to the table among other things.

JOHN MELLEY: Well, thank you very much for sharing your thoughts with us.

TOM: Well, you're quite welcome. It's my privilege.

JOHN MELLEY: Doctor, two for two.

DR. DANA DAY: Well, it must be my lucky day. I should go out and buy lottery ticket.

JOHN MELLEY: I don't know if it's luck. I think it's probably because you've worked really hard and you know what you're doing. [Laughter]

DR. DANA DAY: I'd like to think so.

JOHN MELLEY: You know, I'm sure there are folks listening to our conversation today. They may want to learn more. If they do, what's the best way for them to get in touch with you?

DR. DANA DAY: They can contact our office at (602) 265-9000 or visit our website at AZBalanceandHearing.com.

JOHN MELLEY: The number is (602) 265-9000. And the web address is AZBalanceAndHearing.com?

DR. DANA DAY: Yes.

JOHN MELLEY: Yeah, right. How would you say that your practice is different from other hearing practices in your area?

DR. DANA DAY: The primary way that we are different is we specialize in different areas and we bring those specialties together for the good and the benefit of our patients. Those that have hearing loss due to other issues maybe a concussion or traumatic brain injury and they may need help beyond just the hearing loss. We have a physical therapist that we work with. We have a tinnitus specialist who does a phenomenal job in helping the tinnitus suffer regain control of their life because they literally feel out of control. They have no control over the ringing.

And we have specialists who do balance. And we also have one that does auditory processing evaluations which is how do we process auditory information in the brain. So, we are what we call multispecialty or multidiscipline but it's all for the good of the patient. So, I might see someone, my colleague might see another one, we may fix one problem but know that they need to go somewhere else and so we make sure that they get what they need or they get the services they need. We are very unique in that respect. And I'm very proud of the people that I have surrounded myself with. They are very wonderful at what they do and very loving and caring.

JOHN MELLEY: That's great. Who is your practice not for? I mean if—who is this not going to be a good fit?

DR. DANA DAY: Probably not the person that is just looking for a quick, fast, inexpensive solution to their hearing health issues or balance health issues. One that once they're walking off the street and get something that they could purchase at a drug store. It really has to be a motivated patient that wants to work with us and understands that this is a relationship that we build because again, as I mentioned we cover the hearing aids for the life of the hearing aids. So there is that relationship that needs to be built and cultivated over that time and not a one and done type of appointments.

JOHN MELLEY: Yeah. If there's anything that this conversation has shed light on is that it's not as simple as one stop shop or one-size-fits-all answer for everybody. It—this is a person to person individual treatment program and you need the right people to be able to deal with it.

DR. DANA DAY: Absolutely.

JOHN MELLEY: What's the phone number again, please?

DR. DANA DAY: (602) 265-9000.

JOHN MELLEY: And the web address is?

DR. DANA DAY: AZBalanceAndHearing.com.

JOHN MELLEY: That's great. If there is one message you want to leave with our listeners today, what would that be?

DR. DANA DAY: The one message that I would leave with you is it's time to get your hearing checked. It's time to just become knowledgeable of what's going on. Knowledge is such a powerful tool. Once you know then you can make the decisions on what needs to be done. But if you never know, you sit in isolation, you sit by yourself and you would become less and less engaged with your community. You want to stay active, you want to stay vibrant. If you think you have a hearing problem, find an audiologist, get your hearing checked. If you have questions, give us a call, go on our webpage. We'll happily answer any questions that you might have. But you need to take that step.

Take that step towards better hearing and health. Our line here is "better balance, better hearing, better life." We believe it and we strongly feel that everyone can have a great life no matter if they're five or 95.

JOHN MELLEY: There you go. And I will just say this. I'm pretty sure you're hearing test is probably similar to what I went through. And first of all, it's kind of fun. And second of all, it's totally painless.

And I will admit that the results for me were a little disappointing like I said earlier, but then as you said, knowledge is power and then you can make the decision from there. And why not know? It's your own head why wouldn't you want to know what's going on inside it, right?

DR. DANA DAY: Absolutely. Absolutely.

JOHN MELLEY: You own it, don't be afraid of it. It's yours. Anyway, Doctor, this has been a fantastic conversation. I have learned so much. I have gone through the experience myself but just sitting here and talking with you today, I've added to my knowledge and I want to thank you for that.

DR. DANA DAY: Thank you very much for having me on today. Thank you to the listeners who are listening. And please, if you think you have a hearing loss, check it out.

BIBLIOGRAPHY

THE SCIENCE BEHIND EVERYTHING YOU READ IN THIS BOOK

THIS BOOK IS THE RESULT OF MY 20+ YEARS IN HEARING HEALTH CARE. In this time, I have amassed information from my research, reading of scientific publications, in the classroom (as student and teacher), and from directly interacting with patients' and their loved ones. Below is a list of references that helped me put together this book and present the information to you in a succinct manner. You can access these manuscripts on Google Scholar and/or Pubmed.

"Active Ageing: A Policy Framework." *The Aging Male* 5, no. 1 (2002), 1-37.

Adult Cognition and Hearing Aids. U of Canterbury. Communication Disorders, 2015.

Agmon, Maayan, Limor Lavie, and Michail Doumas. "The Association between Hearing Loss, Postural Control, and Mobility in Older Adults: A Systematic Review." *Journal of the American Academy of Audiology* 28, no. 6 (2017), 575-588.

"Association of Hearing Impairment and Subsequent Driving Mobility in Older Adults." *The Gerontologist* 55, no. Suppl_2 (2015), 137-138.

Bainbridge, Kathleen E., Howard J. Hoffman, and Catherine C. Cowie. "Diabetes and Hearing Impairment in the United States: Audiometric Evidence from the National Health and Nutrition Examination Survey, 1999 to 2004." *Annals of Internal Medicine* 149, no. 1 (2008), 1.

Bassuk, Shari S., Thomas A. Glass, and Lisa F. Berkman. "Social Disengagement and Incident Cognitive Decline in Community-Dwelling Elderly Persons." *Annals of Internal Medicine* 131, no. 3 (1999), 165.

Bernabei, Roberto, Ubaldo Bonuccelli, Stefania Maggi, Alessandra Marengoni, Alessandro Martini, Maurizio Memo, Sergio Pecorelli, Andrea P. Peracino, Nicola Quaranta, and Roberto Stella. "Hearing loss and cognitive decline in older adults: questions and answers." *Aging Clinical and Experimental Research* 26, no. 6 (2014), 567-573.

Burns, Elizabeth R., Judy A. Stevens, and Robin Lee. "The direct costs of fatal and non-fatal falls among older adults — United States." *Journal of Safety Research* 58 (2016), 99-103.

Cardin, Velia. "Effects of Aging and Adult-Onset Hearing Loss on Cortical Auditory Regions." *Frontiers in Neuroscience* 10 (2016).

Cass, SP. "Alzheimer's Disease and Exercise: A Literature Review." *Curr. Sports Med. Rep*, February 16, 2017.

Chen, David S., Dane J. Genther, Joshua Betz, and Frank R. Lin. "Association Between Hearing Impairment and Self-Reported Difficulty in Physical Functioning." *Journal of the American Geriatrics Society* 62, no. 5 (2014), 850-856.

Chia, Ee-Munn, Jie J. Wang, Elena Rochtchina, Robert R. Cumming, Philip Newall, and Paul Mitchell. "Hearing Impairment and Health-Related Quality of Life: The Blue Mountains Hearing Study." *Ear and Hearing* 28, no. 2 (2007), 187-195.

Collins, John G. "Prevalence of Selected Chronic Conditions: United States, 1983-85." *PsycEXTRA Dataset* (n.d.).

Davidson, JGS. "Older Adults With a Combination of Vision and Hearing Impairment Experience Higher Rates of Cognitive Impairment, Functional Dependence, and Worse Outcomes Across a Set of Quality Indicators." Last modified August 1, 2017.

De Leon, M. J., S. DeSanti, R. Zinkowski, P. D. Mehta, D. Pratico, S. Segal, C. Clark, D. Kerkman, J. DeBernardis, and J. Li. "MRI and CSF studies in the early diagnosis of Alzheimer's disease." *Journal of Internal Medicine* 256, no. 3 (2004), 205-223.

Deal, Jennifer A., Josh Betz, Kristine Yaffe, Tamara Harris, Elizabeth Purchase-Helzner, Suzanne Satterfield, Sheila Pratt, Nandini Govil, Eleanor M. Simonsick, and Frank R. Lin. "Hearing Impairment and Incident Dementia and Cognitive Decline in Older Adults: The Health ABC Study." *The Journals of Gerontology Series A: Biological Sciences and Medical Sciences*, 2016, glw069.

"Dementia Prevention, Intervention, and Care." *Lancet*, July 19, 2017.

Desjardins, Jamie L. "Analysis of Performance on Cognitive Test Measures Before, During, and After 6 Months of Hearing Aid Use: A Single-Subject Experimental Design." *American Journal of Audiology* 25, no. 2 (2016), 127.

Ferreira, Lidiane M., Alberto N. Ramos, and Eveline P. Mendes. "Characterization of tinnitus in the elderly and its possible related disorders." *Brazilian Journal of Otorhinolaryngology* 75, no. 2 (2009), 249-255.

Genther, Dane J., Joshua Betz, Sheila Pratt, Kathryn R. Martin, Tamara B. Harris, Suzanne Satterfield, Douglas C. Bauer, Anne B. Newman, Eleanor M. Simonsick, and Frank R. Lin. "Association Between Hearing Impairment and Risk of Hospitalization in Older Adults." *Journal of the American Geriatrics Society* 63, no. 6 (2015), 1146-1152.

Gibrin, PC, AN Ramos Junior, and EP Mendes. "Prevalence of Tinnitus Complaints and Probable Association with Hearing Loss, Diabetes Mellitus and Hypertension in Elderly." *Codas*, 2013.

Gispen, Fiona E., David S. Chen, Dane J. Genther, and Frank R. Lin. "Association

Between Hearing Impairment and Lower Levels of Physical Activity in Older Adults." *Journal of the American Geriatrics Society* 62, no. 8 (2014), 1427-1433.

Govender, SM, CD Govender, and G. Matthews. "Cochlear Function in Patients with Chronic Kidney Disease." *South African/Commun Diord*, December 2013.

Haan, Mary N. "Can Social Engagement Prevent Cognitive Decline in Old Age?" *Annals of Internal Medicine* 131, no. 3 (1999), 220.

"Hearing Impairment and Frailty in English Community-Dwelling Older Adults: A 4-Year Follow-Up Study." *The Gerontologist* 56, no. Suppl_3 (2016), 319-319.

"Hearing Loss and Cognitive Decline in Older Adults." *JAMA Internal Medicine*, February 25, 2013.

"The Impact of Hearing Loss on Quality of Life in Older Adults." *Gerontologist*, October 2003.

"The Impact of Hearing Loss on quality of Life in Older Adults." *Gerontologist*, October 2003.

"An Introduction to MarkeTrak IX: A New Baseline for the Hearing Aid Market." *Hearing Review*, May 15, 2015.

Jacoby, R., and R. Levy. "CT Scanning and the Investigation of Dementia: A Review." *J.R. Soc. Med*, May 1980.

Jamaldeen, Jishana, Aneesh Basheer, Akhil Sarma, and Ravichandran Kandasamy. "Prevalence and patterns of hearing loss among chronic kidney disease patients undergoing haemodialysis." *australasian medical journal*, 2015, 41-46.

Kamil, Rebecca J., Lingsheng Li, and Frank R. Lin. "Association between Hearing Impairment and Frailty in Older Adults." *Journal of the American Geriatrics Society* 62, no. 6 (2014), 1186-1188.

Kelley, Amy S., Kathleen McGarry, Rebecca Gorges, and Jonathan S. Skinner. "The Burden of Health Care Costs for Patients With Dementia in the Last 5 Years of Life." *Annals of Internal Medicine* 163, no. 10 (2015), 729.

Kochkin, Sergei. "MarkeTrak VII." *The Hearing Journal* 60, no. 4 (2007), 24-51.

Lambert, Justin, Rouzbeh Ghadry-Tavi, Kate Knuff, Marc Jutras, Jodi Siever, Paul Mick, Carolyn Roque, Gareth Jones, Jonathan Little, and Harry Miller. "Targeting functional fitness, hearing and health-related quality of life in older adults with hearing loss: Walk, Talk 'n' Listen, study protocol for a pilot randomized controlled trial." *Trials* 18, no. 1 (2017).

Le Goff, Nicolas, Dorothea Wendt, Thomas Lunner, and Elaine Ng. "Opn Clinical Evidence. Oticon White Paper." 2016.

Lin, F.R., L. Ferrucci, Y. An, J.O. Goh, Jimit Doshi, E.J. Metter, C. Davatzikos, M.A. Kraut, and S.M. Resnick. "Association of hearing impairment with brain volume changes in older adults." *NeuroImage* 90 (2014), 84-92.

Lin, Frank R. "Hearing Loss Prevalence in the United States." *Archives of Internal Medicine*171, no. 20 (2011), 1851.

Lin, Frank R. "Hearing Loss and Falls Among Older Adults in the United States." *Archives of Internal Medicine* 172, no. 4 (2012), 369.

Lin, Frank R., E. J. Metter, Richard J. O'Brien, Susan M. Resnick, Alan B. Zonderman, and Luigi Ferrucci. "Hearing Loss and Incident Dementia." *Archives of Neurology* 68, no. 2 (2011).

Martini, Alessandro, Alessandro Castiglione, Roberto Bovo, Antonino Vallesi, and Carlo Gabelli. "Aging, Cognitive Load, Dementia and Hearing Loss." *Audiology and Neurotology* 19, no. 1 (2014), 2-5.

Meister, Hartmut, Stefan Schreitmüller, Magdalene Ortmann, Sebastian Rählmann, and Martin Walger. "Effects of Hearing Loss and Cognitive Load on Speech Recognition with Competing Talkers." *Frontiers in Psychology* 7 (2016).

Melse-Boonstra, Alida, and Ian Mackenzie. "Iodine deficiency, thyroid function and hearing deficit: a review." *Nutrition Research Reviews* 26, no. 02 (2013), 110-117.

Meyerhoff, William L. "The Thyroid and Audition." *The Laryngoscope* 86, no. 4 (1976), 483-489.

Miyawaki, Christina E., E. D. Bouldin, G. S. Kumar, and L. C. McGuire. "Associations between physical activity and cognitive functioning among middle-aged and older adults." *The journal of nutrition, health & aging* 21, no. 6 (2016), 637-647.

Mulrow, Cynthia D., Christine Aguilar, James E. Endicott, Ramon Velez, Michael R. Tuley, Walter S. Charlip, and Judith A. Hill. "Association Between Hearing Impairment and the Quality of Life of Elderly Individuals." *Journal of the American Geriatrics Society* 38, no. 1 (1990), 45-50.

Oh, Esther, Frank Lin, and Sara Mamo. "Enhancing Communication in Adults with Dementia and Age-Related Hearing Loss." *Seminars in Hearing* 38, no. 02 (2017), 177-183.

Palmer, Andrew D., Jason T. Newsom, and Karen S. Rook. "How does difficulty communicating affect the social relationships of older adults? An exploration using data from a national survey." *Journal of Communication Disorders* 62 (2016), 131-146.

Popelka, Michael M., Karen J. Cruickshanks, Terry L. Wiley, Theodore S. Tweed, Barbara E. Klein, and Ronald Klein. "Low Prevalence of Hearing Aid Use Among Older Adults with Hearing Loss: The Epidemiology of Hearing Loss Study." *Journal of the American Geriatrics Society* 46, no. 9 (1998), 1075-1078.

Qian, Z. J., Peter D. Chang, Gul Moonis, and Anil K. Lalwani. "A novel method of quantifying brain atrophy associated with age-related hearing loss." *NeuroImage: Clinical* 16 (2017), 205-209.

Qian, Zhen J., Kapil Wattamwar, Francesco F. Caruana, Jenna Otter, Matthew J. Leskowitz, Barbara Siedlecki, Jaclyn B. Spitzer, and Anil K. Lalwani. "Hearing Aid Use is Associated with Better Mini-Mental State Exam Performance." *The American Journal of Geriatric Psychiatry* 24, no. 9 (2016), 694-702.

Ryu, Nam-Gyu, Il J. Moon, Hayoung Byun, Sun H. Jin, Heesung Park, Kyu-Sun Jang, and Yang-Sun Cho. "Clinical effectiveness of wireless CROS (contralateral routing of offside signals) hearing aids." *European Archives of Oto-Rhino-Laryngology* 272, no. 9 (2014), 2213-2219.

Seimetz, Bruna, Adriane Teixeira, Leticia Rosito, Leticia Flores, Carlos Pappen, and Celso Dall'igna. "Pitch and Loudness Tinnitus in Individuals with Presbycusis." *International Archives of Otorhinolaryngology* 20, no. 04 (2016), 321-326.

Sindhusake, Doungkamol, Paul Mitchell, Philip Newall, Maryanne Golding, Elena Rochtchina, and George Rubin. "Prevalence and characteristics of tinnitus in older adults: the Blue Mountains Hearing Study: Prevalencia y características del acúfeno en adultos mayores: el Estudio de Audición Blue Mountains." *International Journal of Audiology* 42, no. 5 (2003), 289-294.

Snapp, Hillary A., Fred D. Holt, Xuezhong Liu, and Suhrud M. Rajguru. "Comparison of Speech-in-Noise and Localization Benefits in Unilateral Hearing Loss Subjects Using Contralateral Routing of Signal Hearing Aids or Bone-Anchored Implants." *Otology & Neurotology* 38, no. 1 (2017), 11-18.

"Social Isolation in Community-Dwelling Seniors: An Evidence-Based Analysis." *Health Quality Ontario*, August 2008.

Spulber, Gabriela, Eini Niskanen, Stuart MacDonald, Oded Smilovici, Kewei Chen, Eric M. Reiman, Anne M. Jauhiainen, Merja Hallikainen, Susanna Tervo, and Lars-Olof Wahlund. "Whole brain atrophy rate predicts progression from MCI to Alzheimer's disease." *Neurobiology of Aging* 31, no. 9 (2010), 1601-1605.

Su, Peijen, Chih-Chao Hsu, Hung-Ching Lin, Wei-Shin Huang, Tsung-Lin Yang, Wei-Ting Hsu, Cheng-Li Lin, Chung-Yi Hsu, Kuang-Hsi Chang, and Yi-Chao Hsu. "Age-related hearing loss and dementia: a 10-year national population-based study." *European Archives of Oto-Rhino-Laryngology* 274, no. 5 (2017), 2327-2334.

Vignesh, S. S., V. Jaya, Anand Moses, and A. Muraleedharan. "Identifying Early Onset of Hearing Loss in Young Adults With Diabetes Mellitus Type 2 Using High Frequency Audiometry." *Indian Journal of Otolaryngology and Head & Neck Surgery* 67, no. 3 (2014), 234-237.

Weinstein, Barbara E. *Hearing Impairment and Social Isolation in the Elderly*. publisher not identified, 1980.

Yates, J.A., L. Clare, and B. Woods. "You've Got a Friend in Me: Can Social Engagement Mediate the Relationship Between Mood and MCI?" *Innovation in Aging* 1, no. suppl_1 (2017), 1179-1179.

Yates, Jennifer A., Linda Clare, and Robert T. Woods. "What is the Relationship between Health, Mood, and Mild Cognitive Impairment?" *Journal of Alzheimer's Disease* 55, no. 3 (2016), 1183-1193.

Zheng, Yuqiu, Shengnuo Fan, Wang Liao, Wenli Fang, Songhua Xiao, and Jun Liu. "Hearing impairment and risk of Alzheimer's disease: a meta-analysis of prospective cohort studies." *Neurological Sciences* 38, no. 2 (2016), 233-239.

IF YOU READ THIS BOOK, chances are that you or a family member are struggling to deal with impact of hearing loss on your social, physical, and mental well-being. By now I hope you have come to understand the negative impact of untreated hearing loss on overall quality of life and cognitive function.

We thank you for taking your hearing healthcare seriously and for allowing us to provide the education necessary for you to make an informed decision about medically treating your hearing loss.

When you are ready to take the next step to improve your life, your cognitive function, and your hearing health, please visit:

www.AZBalanceAndHearing.com
or call **1(520) 263-8099**
to Schedule a Consultation

Better Balance, Better Hearing, Better Life.

Made in the USA
Lexington, KY
29 October 2019